THE SWOLLEN LEG

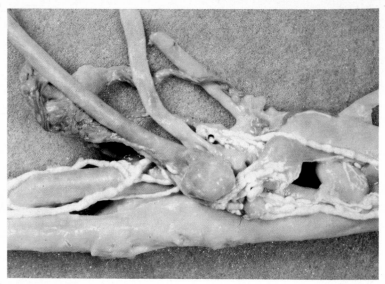

Superficial (red) and deep (white) lymphatics in the groin draining into inguinal lymphnodes. Note that not all nodes are shared by both deep and superficial trunks.

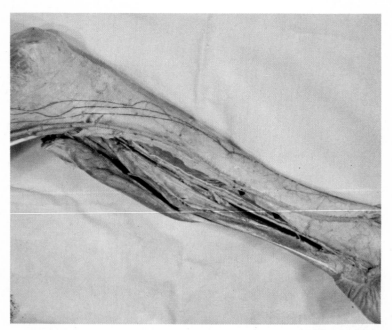

Distribution and course of superficial medial lymphatics (red) in relation to but not in contact with the long saphenous vein and of the deep lymphatics (white) accompanying the post-tibial vessels - dissected by Dr. D. H. Tompsett at the R.C.S., London, cannulated and injected by one of us (J.P.).

THE SWOLLEN LEG

CAUSES AND TREATMENT

H. DAINTREE JOHNSON, M.D., M.Chir., F.R.C.S., Honorary
Consultant Surgeon, Royal Free Hospital, London; Honorary
Senior Lecturer in Surgery, Royal Postgraduate Medical
School; lately Member, Court of Examiners, Royal College of
Surgeons of England; and Examiner in Surgery to London
University.

JOSEPH PFLUG, M.D. (Prague), Ph.D. (London), Lecturer in
Surgery, Royal Postgraduate Medical School, London. Chief
Surgeon, Phlebological and Lymphological Clinic, Göppingen,
W. Germany.

with Foreword by Dr. Karl A. Lofgren, Mayo Clinic

WILLIAM HEINEMANN MEDICAL BOOKS LTD
London

LQMNN J

First published 1975

© H. Daintree Johnson and Joseph Pflug 1975

ISBN 0 433 07042 0

ERRATA

p.77 "Instruments and materials for phlebography." Please substitute Conray 280 for

	Lipiodol	(*item 1*)
	do.	(*item 18*)
p.213	do.	(*line 7*)
p.269	do.	(*line 10*)

Printed in Great Britain by
The Camelot Press Ltd, Southampton

Contents

Foreword

Chronic swelling of the lower extremity is a common disorder, often the cause of much concern to the lay person as an omen of serious disease. Throughout historical times the swollen leg has presented to the physician a frequent problem of correct diagnosis and adequate treatment. The underlying causes are manifold, from benign to serious disorders, from curable to incurable diseases, from acute to chronic conditions, and from systemic abnormalities to disturbances localized in the lower limb. Much anxiety of the patient can be relieved by the physician who has familiarized himself with the basic pathophysiology of the swollen leg so that appropriate advice and effective treatment can be prescribed and performed. Since the swollen leg occurs more frequently in the older age group, its incidence as a medical problem will undoubtedly rise as man's longevity and the world's population continue to increase.

The authors of this book have filled a great need by describing in a thorough and original manner the physical, physiologic, and pathologic changes which so often take place in the lower extremity and give rise to the swollen leg. The differential diagnosis of causative disorders is discussed with clarity and completeness. The varieties of available treatment for the two main categories of venous and lymphatic diseases are described and recommended on the basis of many years of experience by the authors in clinical practice as well as in research. Many refreshing new ideas are discussed, along with older accepted concepts in the mechanism and pathophysiology of venous and lymphatic disturbances in the lower extremity.

I highly recommend this new book as a much needed source of information and guidance to the practising physician and to the surgeon who are challenged daily by the problem of the swollen leg. It will also provide further stimulus to the medical scientist for continued research in the fields of phlebology and lymphology.

Karl A. Lofgren, M.D.

Mayo Clinic and Mayo Foundation
Rochester, Minnesota 55901

Introduction

Swelling of the leg is, of course, a common manifestation of a great variety of disorders, some local and some general. It is with the two main categories of the former that this book particularly deals, namely diseases of the veins and of the lymphatics of the leg. We have chosen 'The Swollen Leg' as our title because it is a physical sign that they all have in common, and because it has been recognized as a clinical entity since before Hippocrates. Recently the French Phlebological Society organized a meeting and published its deliberations under the title 'La grosse jambe'.

In recent years venous and lymphatic diseases have been attracting ever-increasing attention in medical literature; but a great deal of what has been written has not seemed to have taken any cognizance of established laws of fluid mechanics. Treatments have remained largely empirical, or been based on rationales that were, from a physicist's point of view, more imaginative than realistic. Indeed, some of the operations introduced even since World War II have already had to be abandoned.

This book is the outcome of five years of collaboration between a surgical phlebologist and lymphologist of wide experience both in London and on the Continent, and a general surgeon, prematurely retired from surgery, who has spent a number of years since in physical and physiological research. This author was once trained as an engineer, and has a more extensive knowledge of elementary physics and fluid mechanics than is usual among doctors of medicine. The result is a work which is far from a recapitulation of standard teaching. It is essentially thoughtful and critical. But, above all, the treatments recommended have been shown to work.

Our book is divided into three parts. The first deals with normal structure and function. For a proper understanding of phlebology and lymphology a sound basis of fluid mechanics is a *sine qua non*. Of course every doctor has passed an examination in Physics early in his training; but enquiry among our colleagues has established that, while most are satisfied that they must still know enough for clinical purposes, few have in fact remembered even the elements, much less the sort of fluid mechanics needed for understanding, for instance, the requirements and effects of ordinary bandaging. We have therefore felt it desirable to begin Part I with a revision chapter on physics, particularly those parts especially relevant to our subjects. For the sake of simplicity, and to be sure that all our terms have been defined, we have had to start right at the beginning, and hope that not too many of our readers will feel insulted.

The second part is devoted to diseases, their pathogeneses, their clinical features and complications. Methods of investigation are described in detail, with their techniques, indications, contraindications and dangers.

The third part is given over entirely to treatments and their rationales. Surgeons, it has been said, are apt to feel that there must exist a surgical answer to every clinical problem, and to blame themselves if they cannot devise one. We would accept that there have been those who have allowed themselves to be too easily persuaded by facile arguments, often based on unsound fluid mechanics. Their operations have not stood the test of time. We would not wish to stand among Osler's 'last by whom the new is tried'. However, nothing has been recommended here simply because it is traditional, or because others, however famous, have claimed good results with it, or because the rationale has seemed to us logical. Instead, everything recommended has been thoroughly tried out by one of us, and the results followed for many years. For those who like to feel certain they have good reasons for what they do, we have endeavoured to give convincing rationales for what we have found to work, and logical reasons why other operations failed.

In an appendix appear notes or very short essays on subjects related to, but not thought suitable for, inclusion in the main body of the work; or even 'fun' excursions into speculation.

Knowing that many of our readers will select a subject here and there, rather than read through the whole book, and feeling that many of our points, particularly novel ones, call for mention under more than one heading, we have often deliberately repeated ourselves. When such an occasion has arisen we have made no attempt to practise what Fowler called 'elegant variation', preferring instead usually to use the same words over again. We are not unaware, also, of the value of repeating an argument, especially when, being contrary to currently accepted teaching or popular conviction, it may have been discarded out of hand without careful consideration the first time it was encountered.

There has been a distinct tendency among writers in recent years to vie with one another in richness of references, and often to regard quotation of what amounts to no more than a simple assertion by another author as a satisfactory substitute for, or even preferable to, their own logic. It has been tempting to lard our own work with a plethora of references, if only to give evidence that we have read and considered the views of others. However, in the event we have given only those references we have thought might be useful to our readers. In a bibliography which follows this introduction, we have given a number of comprehensive monologues and reviews which in turn give all those references we have omitted to give.

At the time of writing S.I. units had not become widely used in medical literature. Their introduction at a late stage in publication has inevitably necessitated much compromise. The expression '10 mm Hg pressure' should accordingly be thought of as a handy figure of speech rather than as an alternative method of measurement (now 1330 Pa).

One of us holds that without the contribution on basic physics of the other this book would have been more like many others; the other holds that without the clinical and experimental observations of the one there would have been no book at all. Having differed, for the first time, over the relative weights of our two contributions, we have agreed to put our names on it simply in the order they happen to have in the alphabet.

We are especially grateful to Professor R. B. Welbourn, M.D., F.R.C.S., Director of the Department of Surgery at the Royal Postgraduate Medical School, for the way in which he has helped us to overcome difficulties that variously beset us. One of us expresses thanks to Professor J. Calnan, F.R.C.S., of the Unit of Plastic Surgery, for facilities for research; the other thanks the Medical Research Council and the Wellcome Foundation for several years of help during his researches. We both express warm gratitude to our wives, one for the constant physical support she has given him through years of infirmity and her great help with vast technical reading; the other for her toleration of the very numerous absences from home that producing this book has involved.

Finally we wish to put on record our appreciation of the most helpful and co-operative of publishers, and especially of Mr. Selwyn Taylor, D.M., M.Ch., F.R.C.S., whose constant advice and help have done so much to make something out of our efforts.

The illustrations were done by Herr S. Schöllhammer of Albershausen, W. Germany.

H. D. J.
J. P.

London, 1974

Bibliography

Abramson, D. (1967). *Circulation in the Extremities*. Academic Press, New York and London.
(Applied physiology of the venous and arterial circulation of the leg.)

Allen, E. V., Barker, N. W. and Hines, E. A. (1962). *Peripheral Vascular Diseases*. Third edition. W. B. Saunders Company, Philadelphia and London.
(Standard book on clinical angiology.)

Arner, O. (1952). Complications following spinal anaestheais. *Acta. chir. Scand.,* Suppl. 167.
(Theory, practice and complications of spinal anaesthesia.)

Atkins, P. and Hawkins, L. A. (1968). The diagnosis of deep-vein thrombosis in the leg using [125]fibrinogen. *Brit. J. Surg.,* **55**, 825–830.

Bassi, G. (1967). *Les Varices des Membres Inférieurs*. Editions Doin, Paris.
(The aetiology, diagnosis, and treatment of all varicose syndromes, with extensive references and a comprehensive historical review. French.)

Brunner, U. (1969). *Das Lymphödem der unteren Extremitäten*. Verlag Hans Huber: Berne, Stuttgart and Vienna.
(History of lymphoedema and its treatment. German.)

Brunner, U., Kappert, A., May, R., Schoop, W. and Witzleb, E. (1970). *Das dicke Bein*. Verlag Hans Huber: Bern, Stuttgart and Vienna.
(Proceedings of a symposium held in 1969 at Kitzbühl on aetiological, diagnostic, and therapeutic problems of swelling of the leg of venous and lymphatic origin. German.)

Dodd, H. and Cockett, F. R. (1956). *The Pathology and Surgery of the Veins of the Lower Limb*. Livingstone, Edinburgh.
(Widely read and well known, particularly on the Continent.)

Eriksson, E. and Gordh, T. (1970). *Atlas der Lokalanaesthesie*. Georg Thieme Verlag, Stuttgart.
(An excellently presented technique of local and regional anaesthesia. Swedish, German, Spanish, and English.)

Fegan, G. (1967). *Varicose Veins: Compression Sclerotherapy*. Heinemann, London.
(Standard English work on sclerotherapy.)

Földi, M. (1971). *Erkrankungen des Lymphsystems: Grundlagen, Diagnostik, Therapie*. Verlag Gerhard Witzstrock GmbH, Baden-Baden and Brussels.
(A concise and clinically orientated review on all main problems of lymphology based on the standard work by Rusznyak, Földi, and Szabo. German.)

Goidanich, I. F. and Campanacci, M. (1968). *Vascular Hamartomas and Angiodysplasias of the Extremities*. Charles C. Thomas, Springfield, Illinois, U.S.A.
(Extensive description of angiodysplasias.)

Guyton, A. C. (1965). *Functions of the Human Body*. W. B. Saunders Company, Philadelphia and London.
(Applied physiology, with special attention to the physical principles. Guyton is a dependable physicist, but his wording is not always clear to an English reader.)

Kappert, A. and May, R. (1968). *Das postthrombotische Zustandsbild der Extremitäten*. Verlag Hans Huber, Berne and Stuttgart.
(Proceedings of a symposium held in 1964 at Kitzbühl, Austria, on topical problems of post-thrombotic leg. German.)

Kinmonth, J. B. (1972). *The Lymphatics*. Edward Arnold, London.
(Personal experience of a pioneer in this field. Mainly clinical topics.)

Levene, G. A. and Calnan, C. D. (1973). *A Fine Colour Atlas of Dermatology*. Wolfe, London.
(A manual for quick, visual diagnosis of cutaneous diseases.)

Ludbrook, J. (1966). *Aspects of Venous Function in the Lower Limbs*. Charles C. Thomas, Springfield, Illinois, U.S.A.
(Basic physiology of venous system.)

May, R. (1971). *Messmethoden in der Venen-Chirurgie*. Verlag Hans Huber: Berne, Stuttgart and Vienna.
(Proceedings of a symposium held in 1970 in Kitzbühl on latest investigation methods of the venous system. German.)

May, R. (1974). *Chirurgie der Bein und Beckenvenen*. Georg Thieme Verlag, Stuttgart.
(Diagnosis and surgical therapy of venous disease of the leg. Multi-author. German.)

May, R. and Nissl, R. (1959). *Die Phlebographie der unteren Extremität*. Georg Thieme Verlag, Stuttgart.
(Monograph on phlebography of the leg. German.)

Mullarky, R. E. (1965). *The Anatomy of Varicose Veins*. Charles C. Thomas, Springfield, Illinois, U.S.A.
(Monograph on the anatomy of the leg veins, including variations.)

Negus, D., Pinto, D. J., Le Quesne, L. P., Brown, N. and Chapman, M. (1968). ^{125}I-labelled fibrinogen in the diagnosis of deep-vein thrombosis and its correlation with phlebography. *Brit. J. Surg.*, **55**, 835–839.

Nylander, G. (1971). In *Angiography*. Venography of the Lower Extremity, ed. Abrams, H. L. Second edn, Volume II, 1251–1271. Little, Brown and Co., Boston.
(Phlebography up to date.)

Olivier, C. (1957). *Maladies des Veines*. Masson & Co., Paris.
(Standard work on all diseases of veins. French.)

Roberts, V. C. (1972). *Blood Flow Measurement*. Sector Publishing Limited, London.

(Several interesting chapters by various authors on results of Doppler investigations. Very technical.)

Rüttner, J. R. and Leu, H. J. (1971). *Die Venenwand*. Verlag Hans Huber: Berne, Stuttgart and Vienna.
(Proceedings of the symposium held in May 1970 at Zürich. Histology and biochemistry. German.)

Santler, R. (1969). *Zur Verödungstherapie (eine kritische Studie)*. Verlag der Wiener Medizinischen Akademie.
(An analysis of old and new views on how a sclerosant obliterates a vein. German.)

Schdanov, D. A. (1952). *General Anatomy and Physiology of the Lymphatic System*. Medgiz, Leningrad.
(Anatomy and physiology of the lymphatic system. In Russian.)

Schneider, K. W. (1972). *Die venöse Insuffizienz—Pathologie, Klinik und Therapie*. Verlag Gerhard Witzstrock GmbH, Baden-Baden and Brussels.
(Proceedings of a symposium held by the German Society for Angiology at Bad Nauheim, 1970, dealing with topical theoretical and practical problems of venous insufficiency. German.)

Schneider, W. and Fischer, H. (1969). *Die chronisch-venöse Insuffizienz*. Ferdinand Enke Verlag, Stuttgart.
(A monograph on causes and management of post-phlebitic leg. German.)

Sigg, Karl (1962). *Varicen, Ulcer Cruris und Thrombose*. Springer-Verlag, Berlin, Gottingen and Heidelberg.
(Injection therapy. Surgery rejected. German.)

Starling, E. H. (1909). *The Fluids of the Body*. Archibald Constable & Co. Ltd, London.
(Historically interesting but unsound fluid mechanics.)

Tournay, Raymond (1972). *La Sclerose des Varices*. Expansion Scientifique Française.
(History and technique of sclerotherapy. French.)

Yao, S. T., Gourmos, C. and Hobbs, J. T. (1972). Detection of proximal-vein thrombosis by Doppler ultrasound flow detection method. *The Lancet*, i, 1–4.
(Detection of thrombosis in large veins and extensive description of the method.)

Yoffey, J. M. and Courtice, F. C. (1970). *Lymphatics, Lymph and the Lymphomyloid Complex*. Academic Press, London and New York.
(History, anatomy, physiology. Standard work on lymphology.)

The inclusion of an item in this list does not imply that we agree with everything that is in it. In fact, we often do not; and this will be clear from what appears in the pages that follow. The works in the bibliography are mainly what are known as 'standard works' and contain currently accepted concepts, plus much undeniable fact.

Papers reporting increased oxygen tension in blood from varicose veins

Grossman, W. (1926. *Über die Bedeutung regionärer Stoffwechselstörungen für die Entstehung des varikösen Komplexes. Münchn. Med. Wschr.*, **73**, 1432.

Haeger, K. M. and Lindell, S.-E. (1966). Oxygen tension in blood from varicose veins. *J. cardiovasc. Surg.*, **7**, 69–73.

Holling, H. E., Beecher, H. K. and Linton, R. R. (1938). Study of the tendency to edema formation associated with incompetence of the valves of the communicating veins of the leg. Oxygen tension of blood contained in varicose veins. *J. clin. Invest.*, **17**, 555.

Piulachs, P. and Vidal-Barraquer, F. (1953). Pathogenic study of varicose veins. *Angiology.* **4**, 59.

Papers reporting decreased oxygen tension in blood from varicose veins

De Takats, G., Quint, H., Tillotson, B. I. and Crittenden, P. J. (1929). The impairment of circulation in the varicose extremity. *Arch. Surg.*, **18**, 671.

Erb, K. H. and Tiefensee, K. (1931). Untersuchungen über das Krampfaderblut. *Beitr. Klin. Chir.*, **152**, 400.

Krcilek, A. and Brezina, M. (1962). Saturation oxygenée du sang variqueux après station debout prolongée. 1er Congrès Intern. Phlebol. Chambery, Imprimeries Réunies, p. 335.

Paper reporting increased oxygen tension in blood from varicose veins associated with ulceration or severe trophic skin changes, and decreased oxygen tension in blood from other varicose veins

Bassi, G. I. (1956). Rôle des anastomoses artério-veineuses dans la pathologie variqueuse. *Presse méd.*, **64**, 1264–1265.

PART I

Normal Structure and Function

CHAPTER 1

Basic Physics

1. Mass, weight and gravity

Two bodies attract one another with a force proportional to the mass of one multiplied by the mass of the other and inversely proportional to the square of the distance apart of their centres of gravity. When one body is much the larger it is said to attract others on account of its gravity. This is measured in terms of the acceleration it will impart to any object allowed to fall freely towards it. The earth's gravity is $9,81 \times 10^{-3}$ N (981 dynes on the cgs scale). The force with which the smaller body is attracted to the larger is called the weight of the smaller. Thus, while *mass* is the same everywhere, the *weight* of an object varies with its relation to other masses and with their sizes. Since mass is measured with reference to the earth's gravity, mass and weight on the earth's surface are numerically the same. One kg of mass weighs 1 kg on the earth, but about 100 g on a spring balance on the moon, and about three-quarters of the way to the moon it would weigh nothing at all, for the gravity of the earth and the gravity of the moon would cancel out. An object may seem to weigh the same in an aeroplane as on the ground, because it is still about the same distance from the centre of the earth. A few hundred thousands of miles away, the earth's gravity is so small as to be undetectable by ordinary methods.

2. Solids, liquids and gases

Matter consists of unimaginably vast numbers of unimaginably minute particles (and these of even vastly smaller 'particles', exerting tiny electrical forces, and a very great deal of empty space, none of which need concern us here). These molecules (or atoms or conglomerates of atoms) are in constant motion at velocities the mean of which determines the temperature of the material. This gives the particles a tendency to fly apart, which is opposed by the gravitational forces described. For any given combination of temperature and external compression, the particles and forces arrange themselves in one or other of three main patterns, giving the material as a whole the physical properties of a solid, a liquid, or a gas.

In a gas the particles are relatively far apart. In fact they have virtually no cohesion at all. They mingle freely with those of any other gas in the region, and a gas expands indefinitely if free to do so. Gases are also easily compressible, then exerting pressure proportional to the volume they have been compelled to occupy, and to a function of the temperature.

In liquids and solids the particles are much closer together. In solids, except for vibratory movements, the particles retain their positions relative to one another; but liquids continue to flow and to exert pressure equally in all directions. Liquids also mix spontaneously (though more slowly than gases) with most other liquids in contact with them, but form horizontal surfaces with gases and some other liquids. Liquids are almost incompressible, a fact that is made use of in hydraulic brakes. The ease with which liquids flow varies from one to another. Their treacliness, or 'viscosity' as it is called, can be measured (Nsm^{-2}).

Solids do not flow, or only extremely slowly, for even a thin sheet of marble under stress may be observed to bend appreciably in a matter of tens of years, and some solids left in contact gradually invade one another through the years. Many solids are able to undergo varying degrees of elastic deformation, while others are malleable. Some appear to retain their shape until enormous force is applied, when they shatter. Most solids can become dispersed in most liquids to a limited extent, without making any important difference to their viscosity, their solubilities being characteristic for each solid solute and each liquid solvent. Other kinds of dispersion can produce gels, sols, pastes, smokes, and all sorts of special physical states involving complex balancing of little forces.

3. Pressure and suction

Pressure of a fluid represents the weight of bombardment of the walls of a container or of a surface submerged in the fluid, by its hurtling particles. Evidently, therefore, there can be no such thing as a negative pressure. When this expression is used it is 'negative relative to atmospheric pressure' that is meant. Suction is not a pulling force. It is what is experienced when, by muscular effort, for example, a body of air is compelled to occupy a larger space than it did, so reducing its pressure below that of the atmosphere. The atmosphere can then be felt to be pushing into the space. (The lemonade is *pushed* up a straw, not pulled up.) That is why it is impossible to suck water more than about 30 feet high on earth, though there is no theoretical limit to the height to which it can be pushed by an immersion pump at the bottom of a well.

Pressure is measured in units of force per area ($N/m^2 = Pa$, or as dynes/cm^2 on the old cgs scale). Since the pressure exerted at the base of a column of fluid under the influence of gravity is the same whatever the width or shape of the column, pressure may also be expressed as the height of a column of any suitable liquid (mm Hg, cm H_2O). Atmospheric pressure is the weight of the column of atmosphere vertically above a unit of area, and therefore varies according to the altitude at which it is measured. It also varies according to the amount of water vapour that it happens to contain at the moment, that is with the weather. Barometers may therefore also be used as altimeters, provided they are 'zeroed' for weather conditions in the area at the time. At sea level atmospheric pressure is 760 mm Hg or about 101 000 Pa.

Similarly, pressure somewhere in a body of liquid represents the weight of a column of the liquid from the point to the surface, plus the atmospheric pressure at the surface (though for most physiological purposes this atmospheric pressure is neglected. Blood pressure, for instance, is always given relative to atmospheric pressure). Obviously pressure increases much more quickly with descent in a liquid than it does in air. Again, differences in atmospheric pressure with alterations of a few feet do not have to be considered.

4. Hydrostatic pressure

Strictly 'hydrostatic pressure' should mean the transmural pressure at some point in a container of water which is stationary, and in which all forces acting on the water must therefore be in balance. In Medicine, since the word 'haemostatic' had already been appropriated for a different meaning, and since the specific gravity of blood was very close to that of water, the word 'hydrostatic' was also adopted to refer to certain pressures in blood. Hydrostatic pressure at some point in stationary blood, in cm H_2O, could be measured as the vertical distance to its surface in cm. In an open rigid container this would be entirely attributable to gravity. The position of the surface would depend only on the volume of the contents. But in a closed, elastic container, like the vascular system, there is another variable. This is the elasticity of the walls of the container. The stronger this is, the higher the level above which a non-rigid container like the blood vessels, is collapsed by atmospheric pressure (Fig. 1).

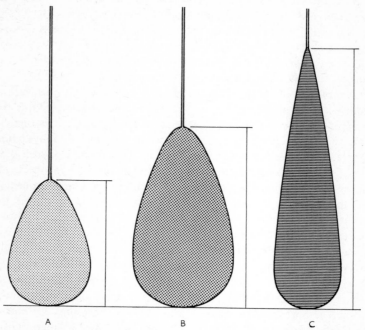

Fig. 1. To demonstrate two ways in which the level above which a closed elastic container is collapsed by ambient pressure, may be altered.
    A. represents a closed elastic container occupied by a certain quantity of liquid and surrounded by atmospheric pressure.
    B. The container and the ambient pressure are unchanged, but the volume of contents has been increased. The level above which collapse occurs has been raised.
    C. The volume of the contents is unchanged, but this time the strength of the elasticity of the container has been increased. Again the level has been raised.

The expression 'hydrostatic pressure' is also used to denote that part of the pressure at some point in a stream of moving physiological liquid, arising from forces which would be present just the same if the liquid were stationary, i.e. gravity and elastic distension of the system. In practice it is measured to the level above which the vessels are collapsed by atmospheric pressure. But it is sometimes forgotten that there is no such level in arteries, and this level should be used only for veins. Also this level does not lie where it would in the absence of cardiac action. When liquid is circulated through a system of tubes by a pump, the pressure at the pump output rises, and that at its inlet falls (Fig. 81, p. 258). The degree of separation of input and output pressures would depend on the relation between the work of the pump and the resistance of the circuit.

So there are several factors which combine to determine the position of the level above which veins are collapsed from which so-called 'hydrostatic pressure' is measured. These are: the blood volume, overall vascular compression, the work rate of the heart and other vascular pumps, and the resistance of the circuit.

Part of the work of the heart maintains a longer column of blood for gravity to act on on the arterial side than in the veins. Part keeps the arteries distended above what would be the 'resting level'. On the venous side cardiac action reduces the basic pressure of the system until it is only just above atmospheric, at heart level. Below this level the veins are distended by gravity, and the level would lie some 30 or 40 cm higher in the absence of cardiac action than it does in life.

5. End-pressure and side-pressure

When liquid moves along a tube it acquires kinetic energy in proportion to the square of its velocity. This kinetic energy has the dimensions of a pressure, and is often known as its dynamic head. At the same time the pressure against the walls of the tube (the side-pressure of the liquid) is correspondingly reduced. This effect is named after Bernouil, and forms the basis for the ordinary laboratory filter-suction pump. End-pressure is simply the pressure (measured in any direction) after the stream has been brought to rest. It is the same as the hydrostatic pressure at rest, and does not include the dynamic head, as might have been supposed. A manometer attached to an end-hole catheter does not precisely record end-pressure when in a moving stream. If facing downstream it registers side-pressure; while facing upstream it records end-pressure plus dynamic head (Fig. 2).

Illustrations in textbooks are apt to give the impression that the Bernouil effect is quite large. But at physiological velocities it is, in fact, small. Even at the speed of arterial blood the difference between end- and side-pressure is only about 1 per cent. To write of side-pressure in lymph (as was done in the newest edition of a multi-volume textbook of Physiology) made odd reading. Even in veins the difference between end- and side-pressure is so small as to be negligible for all ordinary purposes.

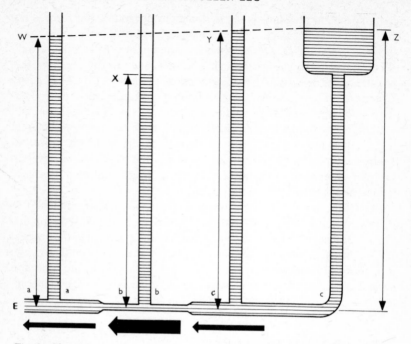

Fig. 2. The end-pressure in the tube aabbcc *is measured by the height* Z *to the surface of the liquid in the header tank. It is the level to which the liquid in the whole system would quickly become adjusted after escape from* E *had been arrested. The heights* W, X *and* Y *measure the side-pressures in sections of the tube with even calibre:* aa, bb *and* cc. *The extent to which side-pressure falls below end-pressure is determined by the velocity of flow (not the volume flow) in the tube* aabbcc. *Where this tube is narrow and flow is faster, the side-pressure is most reduced. There is also a gradient of pressure from* Z *to* Y *to* W *so long as there is flow along* aabbcc.

6. Solid pressure

Since they cannot flow easily and promptly like fluids, solids do not transmit pressure in all directions. But a solid object free to move all in one piece does transmit a force unidirectionally. Moreover, fluid pressure may be applied to one face (as on the piston of a steam engine) and be transmitted through it as unidirectional force. This can be applied to a fluid (as in a syringe) and re-converted into fluid pressure, acting equally in all directions again. If one surface is separated from another partly by elastically compressible solid elements and partly by liquid, pressure may be transmitted partly through the liquid and partly through the compressible solid. For that part of the pressure transmitted through the solid elements in this way the expression 'solid pressure' has recently been introduced (Guyton et al., 1971). Unfortunately a lot of confusion and misunderstanding has arisen, perhaps because the elastic compressibility of the solid was not sufficiently emphasized.

Perhaps an example will best explain what was meant. A syringe has a plunger with a face 1 cm² in area. The syringe is full of liquid and also contains a coil spring. The plunger just rests on one end of the coil spring, and the other end of the spring just rests on the end of the barrel of the syringe. The nozzle of the syringe is connected to a manometer, which records the pressure in the liquid in the syringe (Fig. 3).

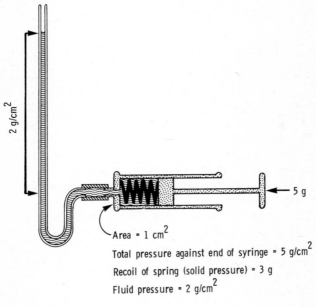

Total pressure against end of syringe = 5 g/cm²
Recoil of spring (solid pressure) = 3 g
Fluid pressure = 2 g/cm²

Fig. 3. Solid pressure.

As the plunger is pushed in, it both raises the pressure in the liquid and compresses the coil spring. The plunger is pushed in with a force of 5 g wt. As the plunger advances the pressure in the liquid rises at one rate, and the elastic recoil of the spring at another. Advance of the plunger continues until a total of 5 g is reached. Let us imagine that this happens when the elastic recoil of the coil spring equals 3 g wt. and the pressure in the liquid is 2 g/cm² above atmospheric pressure. There must be a force of 5 g wt. against the end of the syringe, but the manometer will register only the 2 g/cm² of liquid pressure.

5 g/cm² is what Guyton et al. would have called the 'total pressure'. The 3 g wt. transmitted from the plunger to the end of the syringe through the coil spring (considered as evenly distributed over the whole end of the syringe), is what they meant by 'solid pressure'.

Solids which are not malleable, are all to some extent (though to very varying extents) elastically deformable. Even diamonds bounce off other diamonds. Guyton pointed out that the skin may be thought of as resting on a sort of 'brushpile' of fibres of hyaluronic acid, etc., which transmits some of the pressure of the skin through to subcutaneous structures. In fact there is good evidence that the mobile liquid element of interstitial fluid is at subatmospheric pressure (see Chapter 5: Interstitial-fluid pressure).

7. Osmotic pressure

Owing to the free movement of its particles a solution soon assumes similar concentration throughout. If two solutions of different concentrations are separated by a membrane, and this has apertures which will pass molecules of the liquid solvent, but not molecules of the solid solute, liquid tends to pass through the membrane from the weaker solution into the stronger. The force which drives the liquid is proportional to the difference in concentrations, and to a constant for the solute (and that particular solvent), known as its osmotic pressure. This may be measured by observing the difference of level of the two solutions when the osmotic pressure comes into balance with difference in hydrostatic pressure, and transfer of liquid ceases. Such a membrane is called 'semipermeable'; solids in solution that pass through the membrane are called 'crystalloids'; and ones which will not, and therefore exert osmotic pressure, are called 'colloids'.

Semipermeable membranes are not all alike in respect to pore size so obviously some borderline materials are colloids in relation to one membrane and crystalloids in relation to another. Some membranes, like the walls of capillaries, have pores of varying sizes, only very few of which are large enough to pass some molecules. Such membranes may be freely permeable to inorganic salts, but only slightly permeable to large organic molecules. It would also seem that in capillaries some pores can be stretched to pass relatively large particles like blood cells. It is also probable that the sizes of the pores in capillary walls can change from time to time, according to local requirements.

It used to be suggested that the fluid pressure at the arterial ends of capillaries exceeded the net osmotic pressure of plasma proteins. Rapid extravasation of water and crystalloids therefore took place. At the venous ends the reverse was claimed to be true. Nearly all the extravasated fluids were therefore reabsorbed (all, that is, except any tiny amount that had found its way into the lymphatics). This is why the vascular system is always somewhat distended against its elastic walls, and has what has been called its 'basic pressure' (see Appendix 2).

Though Starling's hypothesis, as it is called, is generally accepted, it obviously is not enough to explain fluid exchanges in the lower extremity of a standing man. For in the capillaries of the feet the pressure at either end must be expected to be 80 or 100 mm Hg higher than at heart level, and must everywhere greatly exceed the osmotic pressure of plasma proteins. A suggestion for a possible mechanism has been made by one of us and is this. When subjected to increased pressure, the walls of the capillaries become less permeable to all sorts of other things as well as proteins. All these would then exert their characteristic osmotic pressures which would easily balance the excess hydrostatic pressure. In fact the osmotic pressure of inorganic salts would more than cope with the hydrostatic pressure in the feet even of a giraffe.

8. Tension. Laplace's law

Tension is a pulling force along a plane, and is expressed as force per length (N/m or dynes/cm). It is such a pity that the word 'tension' was ever used in connection with fluid pressure, for much confusion has resulted. It is true that if the pressure in a tube is doubled the tension in its wall is also doubled, but only so long as the calibre of the tube remains the same, and that must be a very rare event in living tissue. On the other hand, for a given fluid pressure the smaller the tube the less the tension in its wall. The relationship is governed by Laplace's law, which states that, for a tube, $P = T/R$ where P is the fluid pressure in dynes/cm^2, T is the circumferential tension in the wall of the tube in dynes/cm, and R is the radius of the tube in cm. This will no doubt be re-expressed in S.I. units in due course.

To calculate the **longitudinal** tension, the tube is imagined to be closed off by a plane at right angles to its walls and attached to them, so that the pressure on the plane is opposed by longitudinal tension in the walls. The total pressure on the plane in dynes/cm^2 will be $P\pi R^2$, and dividing this by the circumference of the tube will give the longitudinal tension per cm $= P\pi R^2/2\pi R = PR/2$ dynes. But the circumferential tension was PR dynes; so whatever the size of the tube and the fluid pressure applied, the longitudinal tension will always be just half the circumferential tension.

This has obvious relevance to the dilatation and lengthening that occur in varicose veins, and to the relative amounts of longitudinal and circumferential elastic, muscular, and other fibres in superficial leg veins.

Laplace's law may also be used to calculate the pressure which will be exerted by a bandage applied to a limb at any particular tension. Few can have realised how very much less pressure can be expected to be tolerated by the leg of a recumbent subject than of a standing one, and how trivial an amount of tension on an elastic bandage produces a dangerous and painful degree of compression in recumbent subjects.

At a typical ankle radius of 4 cm a compression equivalent to a pressure of 10 mm Hg would correspond to an elastic bandage tension of 54 g/cm. Allowing for the usual 50 per cent overlap, it would amount to 408 g on a 15 cm bandage (only 14 oz. on a 6 in. bandage). Anything larger than this must be expected to interfere with the microcirculation as well as with the venous drainage of the area in a recumbent patient.

A curious implication of Laplace's law is sometimes illustrated to schoolboys as an example of how wrong 'common sense' can be. It is this. Two similar toy balloons are mounted on the two limbs of a 'Y' tube, and air is forced through the stem of the 'Y'. One might have expected that the two balloons would inflate equally together. Instead only one inflates, always the larger, no matter how infinitesimally so. It

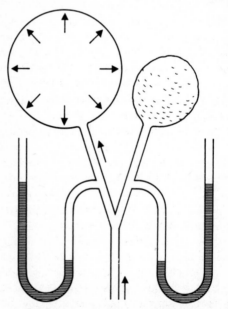

Fig. 4. The Laplacian advantage.

continues to inflate until it bursts, while the other remains flaccid (Fig. 4). When fluid is forced into a system it is bound to find its way to where it will cause the least increase in pressure in the system as a whole. In the one described, the pressures in the two balloons are bound to be always the same. It is mostly because of the operation of Laplace's law that pressure in the system is raised less by forcing a quantity of air into the larger balloon than by forcing a similar quantity into the smaller. Also, the larger the balloon the smaller the *proportional* increase in volume caused by any particular addition to it, and the smaller the proportional increase in tension resulting. Therefore any fluid entering the system is compelled to go to the larger balloon. (The shape of the tension/length curve of vessel wall could be involved in the calculation in exceptional circumstances.)

The volume of a tube of fixed length varies as (radius)^2, and elastic tubes will therefore behave in the same way as the balloons. Thus is blood helped to pass from smaller to larger veins, and hindered from passing from a larger to a smaller one as after a vein has become varicose.

9. Flow. Poiseuille's equation

Just at present 'pressure' is an unfashionable word, and the 'in' word at 'popular' medical level, is 'flow'. It is as well to be reminded, therefore, that although a pressure difference does not imply flow, no flow ever took place without one. The word 'flow' by itself means volume flow; not to be confused with velocity of flow. Volume flow is the rate (in ml/sec for instance) at which a certain volume of fluid is passing across a line or through a plane. Velocity of flow is the mean speed at which the particles of a fluid are crossing a line. The rate of volume flow along a tube therefore equals the velocity of flow multiplied by the cross-sectional area of the tube (Fig. 5).

Liquid driven along a tube by a head of pressure does not all move at the same speed. Provided that it is not flowing at above critical velocity, it proceeds in a vast number of layers each one particle thick, and each sliding over the next outside it. Thus the central layer or core travels fastest; the one in contact with the wall of the tube travelling at zero velocity. This is called 'laminar' flow. Critical velocity varies from fluid to fluid and depends upon such things as the density, the viscosity and the flow pattern. It is calculated from the Reynolds Number. At velocities of flow above the critical level, flow becomes turbulent. That means that it breaks up and becomes completely irregular, absorbs more energy for a given rate of flow, and is associated with noise. It is believed that all flows

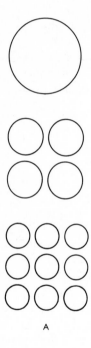

A

Fig. 5. *Each circle represents a cross-section of a tube. In column A the total cross-sectional area of all the tubes in each group is equal to that of the single tube at the top. In column B, when all the tubes in any group are connected in parallel, the overall resistance per unit length of each group is the same as that of the single tube at the top C. In this illustration two vertical veins are connected by three horizontal ones of widths 1, 2, and 3 units. Blood flow will be in the proportions 1, 16 and 81.*

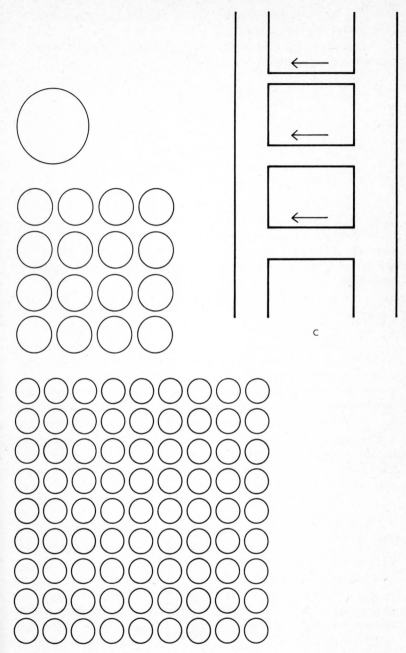

of fluid in the body are at less than critical velocity, except that of blood in relation to the heart valves.

The rate at which fluid is driven along a tube by a certain head of pressure is given by Poiseuille's equation;

$$F=\frac{(P_1-P_2\pi r^4}{8\eta l}$$

Where F is the flow in ml/sec.

P_1-P_2 = the pressure head in dynes/cm^2,
   r, l = the radius and length of the tube in cm.
   η = the viscosity of the fluid in poises

It will be noticed that there is no term for roughness of the inside of the tube, which, of course, makes no difference to laminar flow. A fluid which obeys Poiseuille's equation at sub-critical speeds is said to have normal viscosity characteristics, or to be a 'Newtonian' fluid. Blood has anomalous viscosity on account of its corpuscles, though plasma is Newtonian.

10. Stasis

Strictly 'stasis' means standing still, but has come to mean diminished velocity of flow, and this does not imply diminished volume flow. But most people have a mental picture of stasis which includes a dusky de-oxygenated look, as well as engorgement. Anoxia suggests inadequate blood supply or volume flow in addition to vasodilatation and diminished velocity of flow. It would seem that 'stasis' is a word which has been used a great deal without precise meaning. It is probably too late to try to impose a more exact definition, and so the word is best avoided altogether by those who have something precise to say. We have used it only in the sense of 'standing still'.

11. Syphons and circuits

A syphon is a tubed system, open at the ends but closed between the ends. It is not necessarily of constant calibre. It ends below or exactly level with where it began. Syphons are often described as requiring to be rigid; but there is another possible condition which operates over the greater part of the vascular system. Soft tubes can act perfectly well as syphons so long as the pressure within is always greater than that outside. The point about a syphon is that the energy imparted to the liquid contents by gravity in the downward directed parts of the system either exceeds or exactly equals the energy required to lift contents against gravity in the upward directed parts. In other words the resistance of the system, or the head of pressure required to produce a certain rate of volume flow, is unaffected by whether the tubes run first up then down, or first down then up, or remain all the time on the level.

This makes no difference to the fact that when part of a syphon is dependent the hydrostatic pressure in its contents is raised accordingly. If the tubes are elastic, therefore, they will become dilated in dependent parts, and their resistance reduced in accordance with Poiseuille's equation (Fig. 6). (If any part of an elastic system is elevated the reverse will be expected.) For each vessel resistance is inversely proportional to $(radius)^4$.

A circuit is a system of tubes arranged in a ring. All circuits are also syphons. In addition, so long as the capacity of no part of the system is actually in process of changing, the volume flow of liquid through any plane across the circuit must equal that through any other such plane. The mean **velocity** of flow through any plane is inversely proportional to the overall cross-sectional area of the system in that plane.

In a circuit containing a pump, the rate of volume flow through the system as a whole, as well as through any part of it, must obey Poiseuille's equation. Thus, given a certain pressure head maintained by the pump, a certain overall rate of circulation will become established. The overall pressure gradient must divide itself up between the various segments in accordance with the resistance of each. This sorts itself out cybernetically. If at some point there is insufficient pressure to drive the liquid through the next section at the universal flow rate of the system, liquid will be momentarily dammed up here. Local pressure will rise and the vessels be stretched. Thus will the pressure head and the local resistance adjust themselves to the flow rate, or vice versa.

The volume of the contents of a closed circuit must obviously always exactly match the capacity of the system. Thus any addition to or subtraction from the contents of an elastic system must simply compel a change in capacity. In the vascular system additions to the volume of the blood are virtually all accommodated in the veins, so that a transfusion need lead to no more than dilatation of veins, and not directly affect the volume of venous return as so commonly felt it 'obviously' must. It can, of course, cause an increase in cardiac output, but it does this indirectly through raising venous pressure and through this the rate and extent of cardiac filling. Moreover, how such a transfusion affects venous pressure is as much a matter of venous muscle tone as of blood volume. In practice the **rate** of alteration of volume is found to be of paramount importance (Melrose, 1972).

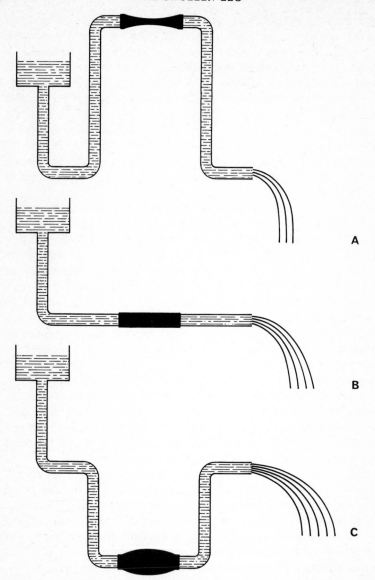

Fig. 6.   A.   *A loop of the syphon is elevated above the header tank. Yet the liquid flows relatively freely. The rubber section is partially collapsed.*

B.   *In this position the rubber section is slightly distended and flow is therefore slightly freer.*

C.   *The loop is dependent. The rubber is distended. Flow is slightly freer again.*

The rate of flow in a rigid circuit is thus independent of the position of the component tubes. The *rate* is determined only by the resistance of the circuit and the work of all pumping mechanisms. In a non-rigid system an elevated segment may be caused to constrict by the changed relationship between tension in the tube wall and the hydrostatic pressure. This can cause increased resistance and diminished flow. Thus elevation, while encouraging absorption of oedema, tends to reduce perfusion of the part elevated.

Syphonage cannot work at all in an elevated non-rigid system in which at any point the pressure outside the tube is greater than that within, for here the tube collapses and becomes closed. Thus a non-rigid tube cannot conduct the 'suction' effect of gravity acting on the contents of the descending section, lifting liquid up the ascending section.

Nevertheless, blood is able to be lifted to the scalp without difficulty, without the aid of syphonage, simply by arterial pressure. Once the blood has reached its destination, been distributed, and begun to return downwards again, it simply falls down the almost collapsed veins, almost as though they were not there. Falling under the influence of gravity, the blood travels at greater velocity than it ascends. Consequently it flows in a narrow stream only requiring a fraction of the available calibre of the veins. These therefore continue to be almost collapsed.

12. Valved systems

In a valveless system like the arterial one, changing from a recumbent to an upright position raises the pressure in all the now dependent vessels the full expected hydrostatic amount instantaneously. Moreover, it will do this whether the fluid in the vessels is stationary or moving. In a system with valves, like the venous one, this is not always so. So long as an adequate head of pressure is maintaining steady flow, and a complete row of valves is open, full hydrostatic effects will be observed. But if, for any reason, the vis-a-tergo fails even momentarily, the dynamic head is quickly expended and flow is halted. The fluid then settles back against the valves which immediately close, then supporting the column and preventing retrograde flow. The column of blood in the venous system no longer constitutes a continuous one all the way to the heart. Instead it is broken up into a number of short intervalve segments. The hydrostatic pressure at any point is now determined by the distance only to the next closed valve in the upward direction. But subsequently blood must accumulate and cannot re-establish circulation until the full 'hydrostatic' level has been reached.

In the lymphatic system, flow at its fastest is extremely slow, and is always from segment to segment. Moreover, lymphatic vessels are closely valved, with all the valves directing flow centripetally. Accordingly lymph displays no hydrostatic effects when a subject stands. In fact lymph pressures are found to be higher in more proximal vessels than in more distal ones.

CHAPTER 2

The Anatomy of the Veins and Lymphatics

THE VEINS

The larger veins of the leg are arranged in two layers, superficial and deep, separated by the deep fascia. The superficial drains into the deep by the two main superficial channels, by a limited number of very small veins called perforators (because they perforate the deep fascia) and probably mainly by the vast numbers of tiny vessels of the microcirculation. These show no sign of division into layers. The two main superficial veins, the long and short saphenous, also pass through the deep fascia to enter the common femoral and popliteal veins respectively.

The smaller, more peripheral veins are densely interconnected and free from valves. The blood in them can flow in either direction, and has a great variety of alternative routes, according to the pressure gradient ruling at the moment. An enormous number of such tiny vessels can be seen in all fascial planes and passing through these fasciae. Most veins over about 2 mm in diameter do have valves directing flow towards the heart and, in the main, from superficial system to deep. Flow in a vein that is injected with radio-opaque medium is seen always to follow the same pattern of veins, being prevented from entering other veins either by adverse pressure gradient or, at this level of size, by closed valves. But valves are active muscular structures with a nerve supply. It is far from certain that in some circumstances they do not actively open.

The saphenous veins

The long saphenous vein starts in front of the medial malleolus, and runs the whole length of the leg on the medial side, outside the deep fascia. It passes behind the medial condyle of the femur (Fig. 7). Continuing its nearly straight course it meets the line of the common femoral vessels obliquely and to their medial side, turning backwards and

21

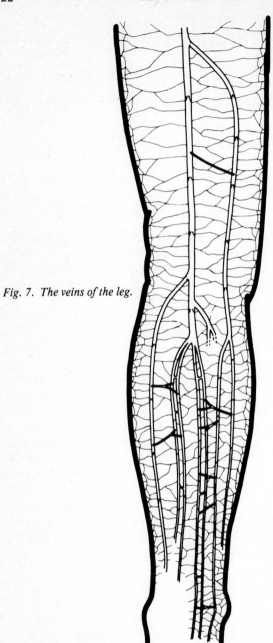

Fig. 7. The veins of the leg.

slightly laterally to enter the common femoral vein. To do this, it must pass through the deep fascia. Here there is an oval defect in the fascia lata, called the fossa ovalis. This contains a thin membrane called the fascia cribrosa. The upper, lateral and lower edges of the fossa ovalis are well marked and easily found. The sheet of fascia forming the medial side does not have an edge. Instead, it passes laterally on the pectineus muscle, deep to the femoral sheath, to which it is attached. The fascia forming the distinct upper, lateral, and lower margins is adherent more laterally to the *front* of the femoral sheath. Thus the fascia lata is in two layers here. The superficial layer is fused with the inguinal ligament and attached to the pubic bone and the anterior superior spine of the ileum. The deep layer covers the muscles.

The short saphenous vein begins *behind* the lateral malleolus, and ascends subcutaneously over the mid-line of the calf. It penetrates the deep fascia at an inconstant level, about at the lower end of the bulky muscle mass of the calf. It enters the popliteal vein just medial to the tibial nerve, most commonly 1 to 2 cm below the line of articulation of the knee. In 15 per cent of cases the short saphenous vein terminates in the thigh, by perforating the fascia lata to enter the superficial femoral vein, or by joining the long saphenous. In 10 per cent it ends in the posterior tibial via an indirect perforator, or by joining the long saphenous in the lower leg. On the average there are 6 valves in the short saphenous vein, and about 9 in the long.

The deep system

The deep system sooner or later receives all the blood from the superficial tissues, as well as that from subfascial structures. Deep veins all accompany arteries, sharing a fibrous sheath with them, with a deep lymphatic trunk, and with nerves. Most medium-sized deep veins are duplicated—the intercommunicating venae commitantes.

The main deep veins of the lower leg are the anterior and posterior tibials and the peroneals. The peroneal veins join the posterior tibials at the lower border of the popliteus muscle. The anterior tibial veins are the continuation of the venae commitantes of the dorsalis pedis artery. Below the lateral condyle of the tibia they turn backwards, through the interosseous membrane to enter the posterior tibial veins, which then become the single popliteal vein. This runs the length of the popliteal fossa, the popliteal artery lying deep to it, and the nerve superficial. It receives the short saphenous vein usually as it lies between the femoral condyles.

The whole neurovascular bundle inclines a little from lateral to medial, and forwards in relation to the femur, from the lower end to the upper of the fossa. Accordingly, it meets the adductor magnus insertion. The vessels, but not the nerve, pass through this into the anterior compartment of the thigh. Here they occupy Hunter's or the adductor canal and become the superficial femoral vessels. After a few cm the superficial femoral vein is joined from behind by the profunda femoris. In a few more cm they unite to become the common femoral vein. At first the artery lies antero-medial to the vein (superficial to it from the front). But in Scarpa's or the femoral triangle the vein passes still deep to the artery and comes to lie on its medial side. The common femoral vein receives the long saphenous vein and passes under the inguinal ligament in the middle compartment of the femoral sheath. The lateral compartment corresponds to a point midway between the anterior superior spine and the symphysis pubis. It contains the common femoral artery. The medial compartment contains only some fat and a lymph gland or two. It is also where a femoral hernia is found. The femoral nerve lies several cm further to the lateral side of the sheath.

As it enters the abdomen the common femoral vein becomes the external iliac. The other main drainage channel from the lower limb is the internal iliac or hypogastric. This receives blood from the buttock, the perineum, and the deeper tissues in the back of the thigh. The precise course and relations of the named veins will not be repeated here. Instead, we shall deal in greater detail with connections between the superficial and deep systems, with valves, and with permitted directions of flow, all of which are of paramount clinical importance, but are apt to receive scanty attention in anatomy textbooks. These will be considered region by region.

The foot

There are two venous arches in the foot, a superficial and a deep. The superficial arch lies subcutaneously on the dorsum of the foot a few cm proximal to the bases of the toes. It receives blood from the toes, and embraces an interconnected network of subcutaneous veins. It communicates with the posterior tibial veins via perforating veins below both malleoli, and with other deep veins in the foot. These perforators in most people contain each a valve directing blood outwards from deep to superficial veins (the reverse of what is usual elsewhere). The superficial arch extends backwards as the superficial marginal veins, which become the saphenous veins, the long in front of the medial malleolus and the short behind the lateral malleolus. The only other valves found in the foot are in these two marginal veins, 2 or 3 in the lateral and 1 or 2 in the medial.

The deeper plantar arch lies in an oblique, almost vertical position, extending about as far forward as the neck of the second metatarsal bone. At its lateral end it lies deep to the flexor digitorum brevis muscle, and the plantar aponeurosis. Almost at once it turns obliquely across the instep, with the lateral plantar artery and nerve, to reach the medial side of the heel. Here it becomes the posterior tibial vein, behind the medial malleolus. The smaller, medial end of the arch plunges deeply into the foot, and passes between the first and second metatarsals to anastomose with the venae commitantes of the dorsalis pedis artery, and becomes the anterior tibial veins. The lateral end of the plantar arch also gives rise to the peroneal vein.

The lower leg

The superficial tissues of the front of the lower leg are drained by the long saphenous vein, most often via a relatively large anterior tributary, supplemented by 2 or 3 smaller ones in the upper part, but occasionally the relative sizes are reversed. The lateral aspect of the lower leg is also drained by short veins which enter indirect perforating veins arranged in 2 or 3 longitudinal rows on the lateral aspect of the calf. The lower and middle thirds of the posterior aspect of the lower leg are drained by the short saphenous vein, via several short tributaries or a single longer one. The upper third of the posterior aspect and the medial aspect drain into the long saphenous and its long posterior tributary. Some of the blood of the lower third of the medial aspect drains into the 2 or 3 direct perforators that leave the long saphenous vein in this region. Some of these each contain 1 or 2 valves directing flow inwards from superficial veins to deep. Every other one has no valves at all; however, and exceptionally, a valve is found pointing the other way.

Subcutaneously on the back of the calf is a constant large vein connecting the long and the short saphenous veins. Usually, in normal people, this contains a valve or two, allowing flow only from the long to short. Occasionally these valves point the other way. In this case, the short saphenous vein is a tributary of the long and has a relatively narrow communication with the popliteal vein. This arrangement is much more common in varicose vein subjects. Sometimes on the medial aspect of the knee a few veins are found which drain straight through the popliteal fascia into the popliteal vein. Similarly, 1 or 2 veins below the patella on the lateral side, pass through the deep fascia into the anterior tibial vein.

The main deep veins of the lower leg are paired and the members of each pair intercommunicate. Just above the ankle the pairs are also interconnected. They have many valves but the communicating channels are valveless. However, there are always valves in the main veins just below where a communicating vessel enters. No further connections with the anterior tibials are found above this, but there are 3 to 6 more between the posterior tibials and the peroneals.

In the soleus and gastrocnemius muscles of man (though not of quadrupeds) there are a large number of longitudinally-running, wide, thin-walled, valveless veins known as venous sinusoids. They are gathered into 6 or 7 collecting channels which drain into the posterior tibial, peroneal or popliteal veins (but not the anterior tibial). These sinusoids are part of the calf-pump mechanism, and there must be periods when the blood in them is completely stagnant. They are the commonest site for a deep thrombosis to start (a condition which rarely involves the anterior tibial vein). Other intramuscular veins in the calf as well as veins in other muscles all to some extent have similar pumping action, but to a much lesser extent; the next most important being those in the sole of the foot. Though valves are rarely found in the calf sinusoids, about one in three of the collecting channels has a valve just before it enters a main vein. The valves in the main vein are also, of course, part of the mechanism.

The thigh

The superficial tissues of the anterior, medial, and posterior aspects of the thigh drain into the long saphenous vein or its anterior and posterior tributaries. The lateral aspect also drains into several small indirect perforators, arranged in 2 or 3 longitudinal rows. Some of the deep tributaries of the profunda femoris vein have passed through the adductor magnus from the back of the thigh, after communicating with tributaries of the inferior glutaeal and popliteal veins. In reverse these form an important alternative route for blood trying to get out of the limb when the common femoral or external iliac veins are blocked. Unfortunately, these veins that perforate the adductor magnus were called 'perforators' many years before the name was appropriated for those, then unnamed, veins that perforate the fascia lata. Other blood is able to leave the limb via microscopic connections with the obturator vein and, when the common femoral vein is still patent, via connections with the superficial veins. The superficial epigastric, the superficial external iliac, and the external pudendal, all of which are tributaries of the long saphenous vein, all anastomose with other veins on the abdominal wall. Many intramuscular veins of the thigh anastamose with others going to the hypogastric and reach the medial and lateral femoral circumflex veins which are tributaries of the common femoral, particularly of the quadriceps femoris muscle. These serve a similar purpose to that of the sinusoidal veins of the calf.

The perforating veins

The perforators have already been mentioned region by region, but for convenience, they will be gathered together again here.

The perforators are short, horizontally-running, very small and thin-walled vessels that connect main superficial and main deep veins (not to be confused with the similarly-named veins which connect the venous systems of the anterior and posterior compartment of the thigh, through the adductor magnus). Most are barely visible to the naked eye, even after injection with Neoprene Latex.

Perforators are divided into 'direct' and 'indirect'. There are about 40 direct perforators in each lower limb, and 160 to 200 indirect ones. The first form a direct link between main superficial and deep veins. The second connect a main superficial vein to an intramuscular vein, and thence to a main deep vein. The direct perforators leave the superficial vein and perforate the deep fascia as a single channel. They then divide into 3 or 4 branches which enter the deep vein separately.

Great clinical importance was first attributed to the perforators by Linton (1938) and later by Dodd and Cockett (1956), who observed that of all the perforators the ones most frequently to become incompetent were those above the medial malleolus, where the results of venous insufficiency are most evident. Indeed, they considered that no serious changes of venous origin ever developed in the lower leg without incompetence of veins in this group. But we hold their importance in normal people to have been exaggerated through failure to appreciate the implications of Poiseuille's Law (see Chapter 1, no. 9: Flow).

All normal perforators are extremely fine, and for a given pressure gradient must carry but a tiny proportion of the total quantity of the blood passing from the superficial to the deep system of veins. True, all circulating blood has to pass sooner or later through capillaries which are even smaller; but their minute size is compensated for by their astronomical numbers, whereas there are only 200 or 300 perforating veins. Yet after both saphenous veins have been removed, all the blood from superficial tissues finds its way into the deep system without any apparent difficulty and without any obvious change in pressure gradient. It must do this almost entirely via the microcirculation.

It seems evident to us, therefore, that the microcirculation must be much more important, in normal people, than the perforators. The importance of the perforators lies, in our view, in their tendency to become dilated, so that they can begin to carry a more important proportion of the circulation, particularly in a retrograde direction.

There are many fine connections between the superficial and deep systems in the foot. All are valveless except two groups, one just below each malleolus, penetrating almost vertically into the foot. These connect the saphenous veins with the posterior tibial and peroneal veins. In nearly all cases each has a single valve directing blood flow outwards, from deep veins to superficial, which is the reverse from what is usual elsewhere.

Above the ankle there are two more groups of perforators connecting the saphenous veins and the main tributaries of the long, with the same deep veins, 2 to 4 on the lateral side, 3 to 5 on the medial. These also contain valves, but nearly always directed the more usual way, from superficial to deep. Occasionally the most distal of these has its valve reversed, like the others just below it. The group above the medial malleolus which underlie the vulnerable 'gaiter' area, are known as 'Cockett's ankle perforator system'. Cockett maintains that every venous ulcer is associated with incompetence of one or more of this group.

In the thigh there are sometimes, but not always, 1 or 2 direct perforating veins connecting the long saphenous vein with the (sub-fascial) superficial femoral vein. All the rest of the perforators are too small and inconstant to justify description.

ANATOMY OF THE LYMPHATIC SYSTEM IN THE LEG

The lymphatics of the leg, like the main veins, are divided into superficial and deep systems by the deep fascia.

Anastomoses between lymphatics and veins or between superficial and deep lymphatic systems (except via a lymph node) do not occur in the lower limb. Moreover, the lymphatic system is strictly regional in character. Material injected into one lymphatic trunk fills only that trunk and no other, until the material reaches a lymph node. Only then do other trunks of the same region begin to fill. The division of the lymphatics into superficial medial, superficial lateral, and deep systems is strict, both anatomically and functionally.

The superficial lymphatic system

Superficial medial group

The superficial lymphatics consist of capillaries (or initial lymphatics) and collecting trunks. In the skin and subcutaneous tissues the lymph capillaries are even more numerous than are the blood capillaries. The collecting trunks are arranged as follows (Fig. 8).

One trunk or two start from the medial half of the dorsum of the foot.

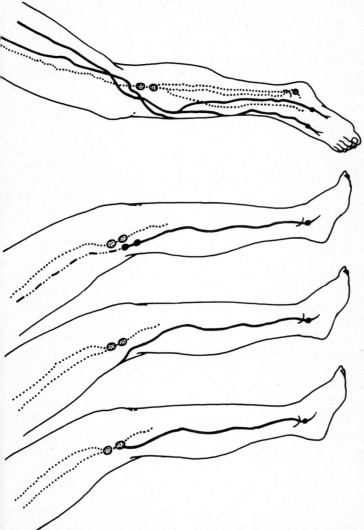

Fig. 8. The anatomy of the lymphatic trunks of the leg. On the right is a single view of the anteromedial aspect of the right leg. There are also three posterolateral view of right legs, showing the commoner variations of the superficial lateral trunk.

These persist as single trunks right up to the groin, following the course of the long saphenous vein, though never in close relationship with it. From the lateral half of the dorsum of the foot a further one trunk or two arise and run proximally on the front of the leg, to join those previously described, just below the knee. Another vessel from the lateral side of the leg passes medially below the knee. All together form a bundle of 7 to 12 intercommunicating trunks on the medial aspects of the knee and thigh. These usually terminate in the nodes of the groin. In about 10 per cent of cases, however, one of these trunks by-passes the groin nodes, going, instead, direct to the pelvic or even the para-aortic nodes. In most textbooks of anatomy the 7 to 12 trunks are called the superficial medial lymphatics.

Superficial lateral bundle

This consists of one or two large collecting trunks that can be identified on the lateral aspect of the heel close to the short saphenous vein. Their courses vary somewhat, but the following are those most frequently encountered:

(a) In about 45 per cent of cases these trunks remain near the short saphenous vein as far as the popliteal fossa, where they terminate in a subfascial popliteal lymph node. The post-nodal, efferent trunks follow the femoral vessels, and end in the inguinal lymph nodes. (In this variety the deep lymphatics of the lower leg have their own separate nodes deep in the popliteal fossa beneath the superficial nodes. In the majority of cases there is no communication between superficial and deep systems, either direct or via nodes.)

(b) In about 20 per cent of cases the lateral trunks remain superficial to the deep fascia throughout the length of the limb, without being interrupted by nodes. Finally they join the medial group of trunks above the level of the knee.

(c) In 15 per cent of cases all popliteal nodes are of uncertain depth and are common to both superficial and deep trunks. The post-nodal trunks then follow the same course as in (a).

(d) In about 10 per cent of cases both superficial (as in (b)) and deep trunks (as in (a)) are present.

(e) In most of the remaining 10 per cent of cases a single trunk accompanies the short saphenous vein to the knee, where it loops back on itself for some 5 cm or so before joining and running with the femoral vessels, as in (a).

The greater part of the lymph of the skin and subcutaneous tissue of the lower limb is drained by the superficial medial group of lymphatics.

Except in varieties (b) and (d), the lateral superficial lymphatics drain only a small area of the foot and calf around the lateral side of the ankle.

The deep system

The deep system of lymphatics drains only the joints and the fascial planes, for there are no lymph vessels in muscle tissue or in bone. The lymph trunks run in close proximity to the main deep blood vessels. They are posterior tibial, peroneal, and anterior tibial. The posterior tibial and peroneal anastomose freely and so form a single functional unit. The anterior tibial lymphatics are entirely separate. In about one in three cases no lymphatic trunk accompanies the anterior tibial artery at all. Instead the deep anterior tibial trunk perforates the deep fascia below the knee and joins the medial superficial lymphatics.

In about 10 per cent of cases the lymphatics accompanying the posterior tibial artery leave it very soon, and follow an ankle perforator vein through the deep fascia. They then join the superficial medial lymphatics.

The lymph nodes of the leg

The popliteal nodes

These nodes vary from one to five in number and are nearly always beneath the deep fascia. However, it is always clear which are serving deep and which superficial systems; for those associated with superficial trunks lie only just under the fascia, while those with deep connections lie close to the popliteal blood vessels. The size, number, shape, and consistency of the popliteal nodes vary so much that no characteristic pattern emerges.

The inguinal lymph nodes

There are often three or four palpable nodes, but there are many more smaller ones which can be displayed only by special methods. All seem to be in superficial tissues. But the superficial layer of the deep fascia is so poorly developed here and the fascia cribrosa so loose, that it is very difficult to divide the area into epifascial and subfascial. A simple method of recognizing deep and superficial nodes is to regard those in close relation to the common femoral blood vessels as deep and the rest as superficial. The number, shape, size and consistency again vary greatly.

CHAPTER 3

The Structure and Function
of Blood Vessels

THE ARTERIES

Arterial blood is distributed in a pulsatile stream at relatively high speed and pressure along vessels that are correspondingly strong, muscular, and powerfully elastic. The pulsatile nature of the pressure head is at present being appreciated to have implications not hitherto suspected which may turn out to have physiological relevance. The distensibility of the arteries is restricted by much less stretchable collagen fibres; but these are corrugated in the unstretched state of the vessels, and do not become taut until the artery has undergone substantial dilatation. It is in the collagen that the chief strength of the arteries lies. In the laboratory the human aorta can be stretched to three times the capacity that it had at zero transmural pressure. That is 75 per cent increase of diameter. It has been shown in life, by Doppler techniques, to undergo changes of calibre of 11 per cent (Gosling et al., 1972). This would imply a 50 per cent increase in volume flow and a $12\frac{1}{2}$ per cent increase in velocity of flow, even without any increase in the pressure head, if blood were a Newtonian fluid.

Plasma does have 'normal' viscosity characteristics, but blood, on account of its cellular elements has anomalous viscosity, though because of axial accumulation of corpuscles, and of a phenomenon known as the sigma effect, it does behave very like a Newtonian fluid in small vessels, down to the size of an arteriole. Even in vessels of the size of a main limb artery, however, blood flow is quite near enough proportional to r^4 for clinical purposes. Accordingly, it should be considered that if the calibre of an artery has been halved by disease, the flow of blood through it for a given pressure difference may have been reduced to one sixteenth of what it would have been at normal calibre.

The smallest arteries, or arterioles, are strongly contractile, and having relatively small overall, as well as individual calibre, offer a pronounced

32

resistance to blood flow. In fact they have the steepest pressure gradient of all the blood vessels. Even in their short length, more than half the total fall in blood pressure of the whole circuit occurs. (Another quarter is accounted for in the capillaries.) Thus, the arterioles play a major role in the control of blood pressure and indirectly, of cardiac output. They also determine what proportion of the blood put out by the heart shall be allocated to each tissue or organ, such as relevant muscles in exercise, or the skin in a subject requiring to lose heat. There are nerve fibres that stimulate relaxation as well as ones that promote increased compression.

An implication of Laplace's law was indicated by Burton (1951), when he pointed out that the tension required in the wall of a contractile tube, in order that it should constrict against a given intraluminal pressure, became less as the tube got smaller. He argued that a small musculo-elastic vessel such as an arteriole while able to constrict progressively with falling pressure, would do so only down to what he called its 'critical closing pressure', when it would become unstable and suddenly collapse completely. His notion is still widely accepted, though it was pointed out by one of us (Johnson, 1967) that Burton's argument required the assumption that the tension in the vessel wall remained the same as its muscle shortened, which seemed unlikely from other experience with muscle. It is our belief that critical closure may occur on occasion, but it is not the invariable logical necessity that had been suggested.

THE BLOOD CAPILLARIES

The capillaries are the smallest blood vessels, varying from 5μ or less, up to 15 or 20μ in diameter ($1\mu = 1/1,000$ mm). According to Poiseuille's equation they must, therefore, offer very substantial resistance to blood flow. In addition, at their smallest size they do not even allow free passage to blood corpuscles without these becoming distorted. The barrier to flow might have been insuperable if it had not been for the compensation of their astronomical numbers, for there are many hundreds of millions of capillaries in the body. (The number of vessels of radius r having a total resistance to flow equal to that of one vessel of radius R, is $(R/r)^4$, while the number of vessels of radius r having the same total cross-sectional area as one of radius R, is $(R/r)^2$.)

Capillaries are of two kinds, the so-called 'true capillaries' and the arteriovenous capillaries, the first halves of which are sometimes called 'metarterioles'. A true capillary consists of a single layer of flattened epithelial cells lying on a basement membrane about 0.1μ thick. These cells are joined together at their edges by a cement substance which may be discontinuous. Channels can often be seen between the cells, and have been estimated to be 40–90 Angstrom (10^{-7} mm; $10^{-4}\mu$) wide. There are many fewer such cannaliculi per micron than in an initial lymphatic, the channels are narrower, and are less readily stretched. In some of the smallest blood capillaries a single cell may appear to go right round the capillary and be joined to itself. The tightness of the junctions, the sizes of the stomata, and with these the permeability of the capillary walls, vary from place to place, from end to end of a single capillary, and probably from time to time as well.

Each true capillary, as it arises from an arteriole or a metarteriole, is surrounded by a ring of muscle, the pre-capillary sphincter. There is no other muscle in the true capillary, or at its venous end. Thus the capillaries may easily be closed off from the arteriole, but cannot be protected from a pathological or gravitational rise in venous pressure.

When a subject stands, the pressure of the blood in any capillary with an open pre-capillary sphincter is bound to rise instantly the full expected hydrostatic amount (80–90 mm Hg). But because of the venous valves, pressure in capillaries open only to venules does not rise at once. Instead, it rises less abruptly as blood is delivered from arterioles, for this cannot pass on into the veins until enough pressure has accumulated to overcome the full hydrostatic gravitational effect assuming the muscle pump has not come into operation.

The pre-capillary sphincters as well as the arterioles contract rhythmically (though asynchronously) as well as being able to contract tonically. Since intracapillary pressure will be substantially altered by whether or not the capillary is open to its arteriole, it seems more likely that capillaries are continually changing their role from that of net exuders to that of net absorbers or vice versa, rather than being always absorbers at one end and exuders at the other, as wrongly supposed to have been suggested by Starling. The muscle of the capillary sphincters and of the arterioles is particularly sensitive to the local levels of concentration of oxygen or of metabolites, or to pH. Changes in these, in one direction associated with tissue activity, and in the other with influx of fresh blood, could explain this rhythmic variation of muscle state.

The whole of a blood capillary used to be thought to be contractile, but this is now denied. However, the very small number of capillaries that appear to contain blood at any one moment, is a conspicuous feature of an inactive tissue. The fact that they become empty when out of use, in spite of the continued level of pressure in the venules, suggests that the capillaries must be at least elastic. This notion is further supported by the crinkled appearance of the cells when the capillary is empty.

The slightly larger arteriovenous capillaries communicate directly between the arteriole and the venule, particularly between their ends.

They have a little muscle in their walls, but no separate pre-capillary sphincter. Many true capillaries arise from the arterial half of an arteriovenous capillary, and others end in the venous half. When an arteriole is open blood from it has alternative routes at each arteriovenous communication. Either it goes by these or it goes by a group of true capillaries. Thus the capillaries tend to form groups or units, with one or more of the shortcircuiting routes. These units vary from tissue to tissue in their internal arrangements. In some each arteriole gives off several arteriovenous capillaries, each of which is associated with a number of intercommunicating true capillaries, all of which finally find their way into a single venule. In another kind, typical of muscle, several arterioles form a ring, and several venules a similar one. The two rings are joined by direct channels of varying length, and also by a number of little systems of true capillaries.

In addition to the tiny arteriovenous communications described, there are in some tissues anastomotic channels joining vessels rather too large to be described as arterioles and venules. Such anastomoses have been postulated for the leg as a cause of varicose veins (Piulachs & Vidal Barraquer, 1953), but none have been reported to have been seen there yet.

THE VEINS

The veins conduct the cellular elements of the blood back to the heart, along with a volume of fluid almost exactly equal to that put out by the arteries, as well as CO_2 and other metabolites for distribution to the various specialized sites for their disposal. Venous blood proceeds at low pressure and moderate speed, along vessels that are correspondingly thin walled and more capacious as well as more numerous than the arteries. In fact about 70 per cent of the blood is in veins at any one time. The veins are therefore often described as the 'capacitance' part of the vascular system, being able to alter the absolute volume of their contents with proportionally less change of calibre, and resistance to flow, than can other vessels. Thus, by becoming only half as wide again, the veins alone can nearly double the capacity of the entire vascular system.

Muscle in the walls of veins exerts tone and is also capable of vigorous venocompression on stimulation of certain sympathetic nerves. There are no relaxor or venodilator fibres. The great veins have other important functions in controlling ventricular filling pressure, and in initiating changes in circulation rate, as well as in cushioning the effects of additions to or losses from the blood volume.

An important effect of the capacity of veins to dilate in response to a small increment of pressure is this. It can be observed during dynamic phlebography of the popliteal vein. As the ankle is extended and the calf contracted, the popliteal vein is seen to dilate quite widely. Say its width were to double, that would mean that its capacity had increased four-fold, and its resistance to flow decreased sixteen-fold. At the same time the tension in its wall to oppose the same pressure would also have had to double. The vein is then seen to constrict down to its former size more slowly. Thus the venous system is protected from the sudden substantial rise in pressure that would have been occasioned by activation of the calf.

The amount of muscle in the wall of any particular vein is proportional to the pressure that it will be called on to withstand. Accordingly, the veins of the lower extremity, which have to cope with high levels of hydrostatic pressure in the upright position, have more muscle than have more proximal veins. The amount of support that a vein receives from surrounding structures is another important factor in determining how sturdy a vein must be in proportion to its size. Unlike the superficial veins, the deep veins of the leg are enclosed within the tough, inelastic deep fascia. Moreover, many of them are also among muscle fibres, as well as being within the individual sheath of a muscle. These sheaths vary in thickness and in tightness, particularly strong being that of the calf muscles, and the particularly capacious and thin-walled sinusoidal veins within these have been mentioned in several connections.

Veins are more distensible than arteries, and dilate in response to relatively small increments of internal pressure. Many more of the muscle fibres in veins, than in arteries, are longitudinal.

When a vessel is neither in process of dilating nor of constricting, the compression being exerted by its walls must be exactly equal to the blood pressure there. The compression which is being exerted by arteries therefore has to be some 10 to 15 times greater than by veins of similar size. Yet the walls of veins are much more than a tenth to a fifteenth of the thickness of those of arteries. The same is true of any of the constituent tissues. It may be said, therefore, that the tension able to be exerted in the walls of veins is much larger *in proportion to the blood pressure within* than it is in those of arteries. When a vessel changes its size it has to adjust the tension in its wall proportionately to resist the same presure ($P = T/R$). Thus the veins are better equipped to adjust themselves to altered capacity without alteration of blood-pressure (their 'capacitance' function).

The vasa vasorum of veins are much more numerous than those of arteries, for the veins do not, like the arteries, derive any of the blood that nourishes their walls from their own lumens. Indeed, the vasa vasorum of veins penetrate right down to the intima. Nor do the venous vasa vasorum drain into the lumen of the main vein, but instead are gathered together to drain further afield. An important clinical result of this is that if the blood in a vein clots, the vasa vasorum are unlikely to be affected. The main wall, therefore, survives and can initiate the process of vascularization of the thrombus, and re-canalization of the vein.

While arteries intercommunicate only to a very limited extent, veins intercommunicate freely; and while no arteries at all are equipped with valves, nearly all veins over 2 mm in width are so. All veins over this size in the leg have valves, as do abdominal veins draining the leg, except the vena cava. These valves are more numerous in the leg than in the arm, and in the deep veins of the leg than in the superficial ones. Indeed, in the deep veins of the leg valves occur every inch or so. The valves direct blood towards the heart and in the main from superficial to deep systems in the leg. Their function is described under 'The Accessory Venous Pumps'. Just on the heart-ward side of each valve a little ballooning of the vein occurs, which gives most veins a beaded appearance.

Above a level near the top of the heart, where venous blood pressure is equal to atmospheric, the veins are collapsed; and as can be seen just under the skin, so they are in any part of the arm or leg which is held above this level. This does not mean that these collapsed veins are not conducting any blood. The size of the stream of blood returning from the head, for instance, is proportional to the rate of volume flow divided by its velocity of flow. But this blood in the neck is falling quite fast under the influence of gravity. The size of stream that this implies does not require more than a fraction of the available venous calibre. Wherever veins are collapsed, in the leg of a patient undergoing operation in Trendelenburg's position, for instance, air is apt to be sucked into a vein that is opened.

The larger the calibre of a vessel for any given volume flow, the slower the velocity of flow. The word 'stasis' is commonly used for a slow velocity of flow, without any thought to volume flow. There is no doubt that stasis is generally accepted to be something undesirable. It is important to appreciate that so used the word does not imply diminished volume flow in the microcirculation. Perhaps we should be careful to use some other expression such as 'inadequate blood supply' when that is what is meant. This may be associated with *increased* velocity of flow in veins that have remained patent when others have thrombosed.

Valves

Venous valves consist of a double layer of endothelium enclosing a small amount of muscle derived from the media of the vein. Most of them have two cusps, though a few are monocuspid or tricuspid. The cusps are attached to a fibrous ring, which is a less distensible part of the vein wall. Just above each ring the vein wall is thinned by a deficiency of circular muscle, the muscle here being no more than a fifth of its thickness elsewhere. This causes the characteristic intermittent bead-like distension.

Valves are described as 'ostial' or 'parietal' according to their position in the vein. The ostial ones are those which are found just before the vein enters another. In addition, wherever a tributary enters another vein obliquely, a sort of flap-valve mechanism operates, and when a vein is injected with radio-opaque material, no retrograde flow into tributaries is seen, even up to the first cusped, or ostial valve. Moreover, it is impossible to inject simultaneously two veins that join higher up, for injecting one occludes the mouth of the other.

Cusped valves are more numerous in deep veins than in superficial ones, and more numerous more distally than more proximally. But valves are very inconstant in both position and number, even occasionally in direction, both from patient to patient, and from side to side in the same patient.

CHAPTER 4

The Systemic Circulation

THE CARDIOVASCULAR SYSTEM

Added together, the vascular system makes a 6-litre elastic container into which the heart alternately ejects about $\frac{1}{4}$ litre of blood and passively receives back a similar quantity. Because the vessels plus the heart constitute a closed system, their total capacity must always exactly match the blood volume. Any gain to (from the gut, by transfusion, etc.) or loss from it (via the kidneys, oedema, haemorrhage, etc.) simply compels a similar change in the capacity of the container, largely by change of venous calibre. It can have no direct effect on the rate of venous inflow to the heart. It does, however, affect the passive element of basic compression; unless compensated for by a change in the active element, mainly venous tone, it is bound to affect venous pressure.

According to Barron (1960): 'the rate at which blood from the reservoir enters the right heart determines the cardiac output', but this in turn must depend upon the central venous pressure and the resistance of the myocardium to the rate and extent of cardiac filling. The former is actively controlled by venous, and more remotely by arteriolar, tone; both are under the control of the nervous system.

When metabolism in an area increases, the resulting reduction in oxygen concentration, depression of pH, and accumulation of metabolites cause the arterioles and precapillary sphincters of the area to relax and open. So long as cardiac output remains unchanged, this causes arterial pressure to fall and venous pressure to rise. But both these changes reflexly promote tachycardia.

Each diastole begins with accumulated auricular inflow at its peak. As the auriculo-ventricular valves open and blood pours into the now relaxed ventricles, auricular pressure falls and ventricular pressure rises. The rate of ventricular filling therefore declines progressively. During a period known as 'diastasis', occupying about a fifth of the whole resting cardiac cycle, almost no filling occurs. As tachycardia shortens each cycle, to begin with this is entirely at the expense of diastasis. If everything else remains the same, stroke volume is only slightly reduced.

39

Cardiac output therefore increases nearly in proportion to the increase in pulse rate.

However, after the pulse rate has quickened enough to use up the whole of diastasis, further shortening of the cycle begins to encroach on the more rapid part of diastolic filling. Soon further tachycardia can no longer increase output, for decrease in completeness of filling begins to match the effect of increased pulse rate. Further increase in output can now be achieved only with *faster* filling. This demands increased central venous pressure or diminished myocardial resistance to filling. The latter can result from neural stimulation. There is also more complete and faster systolic emptying. The rise in central venous pressure can also be effected by increase of venous tone.

At the same time as promoting increase in pulse rate, a fall in arterial pressure stimulates arteriolar constriction, which is overridden locally by the effects of increased metabolism. The overall result is therefore to constrict arterioles leading to less active tissues. If the increase in metabolism is such that venous pressure rises in spite of tachycardia with its increased rate of cardiac withdrawal, this too will increase the rate and extent of cardiac filling, increase cardiac output, and further restore arterial pressure.

The effects of change of posture

Adopting an upright posture from a recumbent one greatly increases the gravitational or hydrostatic effects on the blood in now dependent vessels. Changes in vascular muscle tone sufficient fully to compensate for this do not occur, and dependent vessels, particularly the veins, become somewhat dilated, while less dependent ones constrict. About half a litre of blood is transferred mainly from the heart and the pulmonary circulation to the veins of the lower limbs. The thighs accommodate the larger volume, but the increase in girth of the lower legs is more conspicuous. Both the end-systolic and end-diastolic volumes of the heart decrease, and, though there may be a slight rise in pulse rate, cardiac output is reduced. The diminution of circulation rate is accompanied by some arteriolar constriction which affects the arms as well as the legs.

Some subjects when they stand up, even from a sitting position, experience a few moments of giddiness, associated with a fall in arterial blood pressure. This is because it takes a few heart beats to effect this transfer of blood. While the leg veins are being filled no venous blood is passed on, and there is a momentary failure of venous return. (In most subjects this is fully compensated for by transitory constriction of great veins which maintains cardiac filling pressure.) Output therefore also fails, and there is a moment of cerebral anoxia.

THE ACCESSORY PUMPS

In addition to its main pump the cardiovascular system has several accessory pumping mechanisms. There is one on the arterial side and five, two major and three minor, which assist circulation through the veins: the respiratory pump, the muscle pump, the pulse pump, one derived from the pumping action of the veins themselves, and what we have called the 'Laplacian' pump. Neither the respiratory nor the muscle pump is essential to the circulation. This is demonstrated by the fact that standing quietly with the muscle pump inoperative, and putting the respiratory pump out of action as well by holding the breath, does not cause any noticeable failure of venous inflow to the heart, or of cardiac output. There is no moment of dizziness, for instance, such as is experienced by some subjects when they stand up suddenly from a sitting position and suffer such a momentary failure.

The arterial pump

The strongly elastic walls of the larger arteries are able to stretch, and absorb and store some of the energy of ventricular contraction, then to return it to sustain the power of continued flow during diastole. This may not be a pump at all, for strictly a pump must put energy into a system. But it is by no means impossible that the muscle of the arteries actively constricts during diastole; indeed there are good morphological reasons for guessing that it very probably does.

The respiratory pump

This may be the most important of the venous pumps, for though its work may amount to no more than the equivalent of lifting blood 10 or 15 cm, many ml are moved for every breath. Moreover, the effect continues all the time, day and night.

During inspiration, with descent of the diaphragm, intrathoracic pressure falls and intra-abdominal pressure rises, so that the difference between them becomes greater. Blood, therefore, rushes from the capacious abdominal vena cava into the short intrathoracic segment and, if the heart is in diastole, straight on into the ventricle.

During this phase, pressure in the external iliac veins may exceed that in the femoral veins, but blood is prevented from being propelled backwards down into the legs, by closure of the valves in the iliac veins. However, blood flow in the common femoral vein is temporarily arrested.

During expiration, intra-abdominal pressure falls and intrathoracic pressure rises, though remaining below either atmospheric or intra-abdominal pressure. Meanwhile, blood has been accumulating in the femoral veins, and the pressure rising. Pressure in them soon exceeds the now reduced pressure in the iliac veins, and blood is propelled into the relatively empty, though potentially wide, veins of the abdomen. During expiration, the flow of blood from the abdominal into the thoracic vena cava is much slowed, although it never stops altogether, since there continues to be a pressure gradient in the direction of the heart. This mechanism could be making a substantial contribution to the work of circulating the blood.

The muscle pump

This is the most powerful, and most spectacular of the venous pumps. But it operates only during exercise of the legs, and only on a proportion of the venous blood. Its most important role is probably in preventing the intracapillary pressure in the feet and lower legs from rising excessively during exercise, and so embarrassing fluid exchanges with active tissues just when these are particularly important.

Though the muscle-pump mechanism is represented to some extent in every muscle, it is in the calf muscles that the most important one is to be found. Not only do these muscles share a particularly sturdy communal fibrous sheath, but also these muscles contain many wide sinusoidal veins that together hold quite a lot of blood (Figs. 9 and 10). When the calf muscles contract, these veins are powerfully compressed. In a normal leg the larger perforating vessels by which some blood might be forced back into the superficial veins, are guarded by valves. Therefore, the blood is compelled to pass into other deep veins, such as the popliteal. It has been reported that enough pressure has been generated to force blood under a sphygmomanometer cuff, inflated to a pressure of 90 mm Hg. This was as high as the hydrostatic pressure in the calf veins of a tall standing man. One would not expect the pressure in the sinusoids of the muscle pump to exceed this, since that is the level of pressure at which the blood would escape freely into other deep veins.

When the calf muscle relaxes and ceases from compressing the sinusoidal veins, the pressure in the sinusoids falls sharply. They cannot be immediately filled from peripheral capillaries; nor, because of the valves in larger veins, can blood return into them retrogradely. Blood can and does immediately enter them from the superficial system. However, it

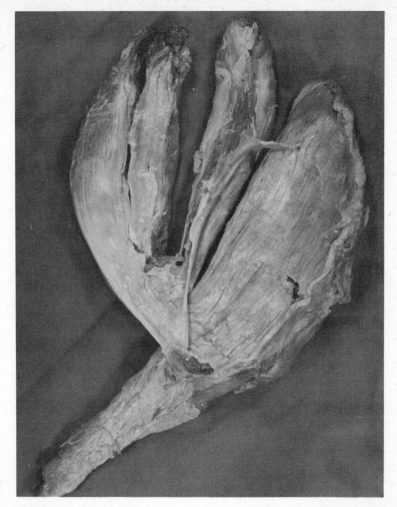

*Fig. 9. A human calf muscle. Unless the veins are properly treated, they collapse
and are not apparent.*

does so via the very limited number of little perforating veins, and via the
vastly more numerous, though individually minute vessels of the
microcirculation, which takes a few moments. More important still is the
fact that the muscle sinusoids are collectively very capacious, and there is
not enough blood in main superficial veins to fill them, and this source of
blood cannot, as it were, 'keep pace' with a continuingly acting calf
pump. Each time the calf muscles relax, the pressure in both deep and

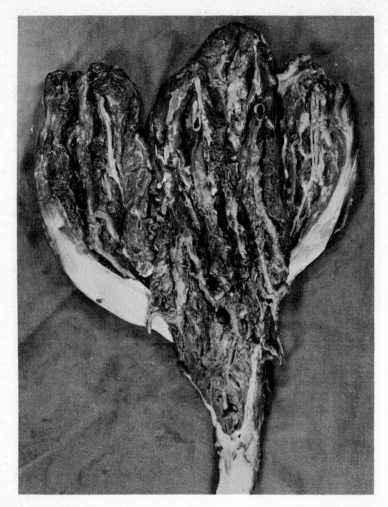

Fig. 10. The veins have been filled with Neoprene Latex. Compare with Fig. 9.

superficial veins falls markedly. When venous blood pressure is measured, as described in Chapter 8: Pressure Measurements, the pressure falls by about 50 per cent.

The pulse pump and spontaneous activity of veins

All the deep arteries share an inelastic fibrous sheath with veins and lymphatics. Each time the artery pulses it raises the pressure in this sheath and compresses the veins and lymphatics. Each time during diastole and fall of arterial pressure, the veins and lymphatics refill. Moreover, on account of their valves, they refill only from more proximally. Thus a pumping action on lymph and venous blood results. The energy for the operation is derived from myocardial action, and constitutes an important contribution towards propulsion of venous blood.

At dynamic phlebography, during activation of the calf pump, each contraction of the calf muscles is seen to be accompanied by wide dilatation of the popliteal vein. This then recovers its former size less abruptly. This recovery is mainly due to run-off; but it is quite possible that each time it happens there is an element of venous contraction. In fact every valved vein in the body could be acting like a little accessory heart.

Laplacian pump

There is a mathematical reason why, if two tubes of similar elasticity of wall come into continuity, the smaller tends to empty into the larger. (See Chapter 1, no. 8.) The mechanism may have an important bearing on the effects of varicosity in superficial veins. The same considerations also help smaller peripheral veins to empty into larger, more proximal ones. We have named this effect the 'Laplacian pump', since Laplace's law is involved.

VENOUS PRESSURE AND FLOW

Venous pressure has often been described as 'what is left of arterial pressure after the blood has passed round the vascular system'. This would seem to suggest that without cardiac action venous pressure would vanish, but this is the reverse of what actually happens at death. For when the heart ceases to beat, arterial pressure does fall; but *venous pressure rises* until the two reach equality at a level several times that of normal venous pressure. This represents the continued squeeze of the blood by inert elastic tissue in the walls of blood vessels. We have found this to be about 18 cm H_2O in the dog. During life when active muscle tone will be added, the total compression must be greater than this. (See Basic Compression, Appendix 2.)

This feature of the vascular system was referred to as the 'basic compression' of the system (Johnson, 1964). Its importance was stressed by Barron (1960) when he wrote: 'The volume of the blood exceeds what would be the total capacity of the vascular system if all the vessels were in a relaxed' (unstretched) 'state'. Starling also recognized what he called the 'mean systemic pressure'.

As described by Bayliss and Starling (1894), arterial pressure represents basic pressure plus the effect of cardiac action, and venous pressure represents basic pressure *minus* the effect of escape of blood into the diastolic heart.

The extent to which venous pressure is below basic pressure is determined by the relation between the total work of the heart plus all the other pumping mechanisms, and the resistance of the circuit. Thus dilatation of capillaries and arterioles tends to **raise** venous pressure nearer to 'basic' level, and increased cardiac work tends to **reduce** venous pressure.

An engineer would expect

$$\frac{\text{cadiac output}}{\text{mean venous pressure}}$$

to be a useful index of cardiac efficiency.

If venous pressure just before the heart were ever to fall below ambient pressure, the veins here would become collapsed, cardiac filling could not take place, and cardiac output would cease. That central venous pressure does not ever fall below ambient pressure has been ascribed to complicated reflexes (Rushmer, 1961). However, as explained in Chapter 1, no. 3, there is no such thing as **active** suction. All pumps are filled by positive pressure from outside. The heart can reduce pressure in the great veins nearly to zero **relative to ambient pressure**, but it is surely obviously impossible for it to reduce venous pressure below ambient pressure.

One commonly comes across the expression 'the force needed to lift the blood from the feet to the heart'. It suggests a failure to grasp the significance of the fact that the vascular system is a syphon or circuit (see Chapter 1, no. 11). The energy required to lift the blood from the feet is exactly matched by that imparted to the blood by gravity on its way down the legs.

Syphon action safeguards venous circulation, but cannot guarantee any particular **rate** of circulation. Like depression of venous pressure, this depends upon the relation between the resistance of the circuit and the work put out by all the pumping mechanisms. In resting conditions the heart alone is capable of maintaining an adequate circulation, but whether it can always manage alone or not, it does in fact have very considerable help from several powerful accessory pumps. Like the heart, these are all valved mechanisms worked by muscular compression. Without these valves they could not make any contribution towards propulsion of the blood. Indeed, to have any effect they must produce enough retrograde flow to close at least one valve in an upstream direction to, as it were, take a purchase against, to be able to give the blood a push in the right direction.

Thus syphonage assists venous circulation everywhere below the level of venous collapse. Above this level syphonage cannot work in the non-rigid veins of the neck, for instance. Blood is lifted to the scalp entirely by the arterial pressure created by cardiac action. When the blood reaches its destination and after carrying out its peripheral function it starts down again in veins. Yet these seem collapsed. But they are not, of course, completely empty. The blood in the veins of the neck is dropping relatively fast and therefore travels in a relatively thin stream. In fact it does not need more than a fraction of the available calibre of the veins. This is why these remain fairly collapsed.

In a system of rigid tubes divided into segments by valves, it is possible to move liquid from the first segment into the second only by displacing an equal volume from the second into the third, and so on, right to the top of the rigid segment. The liquid rising from the first to the second segment in such a system has to overcome hydrostatic pressure equivalent to the whole height of the rigid segment. The pump would also have to impart substantial acceleration to the whole mass of blood in the rigid tubes, and this would use much pump energy.

In a system of elastic tubes, however, liquid may be squeezed from the first segment into the second without need for all these progressive displacements, simply by distending the second segment. The movement of the liquid has to overcome, in the first place, only the resistance to further stretching of the second segment, and much pump energy is saved.

At dynamic phlebography the popliteal vein can indeed be seen to dilate suddenly and widely, on activation of the calf pump, and then to recover its previous size less abruptly. Loss of this ability to dilate is, in our view, one of the most serious effects of deep venous thrombosis.

Mean venous pressure

True mean venous pressure is not simply the midpoint between the maximum and minimum levels during the cardiac cycle, though this approximation is usually accepted for physiological and medical purposes. True mean venous pressure is arrived at by making a graph of venous-pressure/time. The area between this graph and the zero line is measured by counting squares on the graph paper.

Mean venous pressure =

$$\frac{\text{The area beneath the graph of pressure/time}}{\text{The duration of the graph}}$$

CHAPTER 5

Interstitial Fluid

Physical state

'Interstitial fluid', and 'tissue fluid' as it is commonly called in Britain, are both misnomers for what occupies the interstitial compartment; for it is now generally accepted that there is no continuous body of ordinary liquid between the cells, as used to be supposed. In fact, as pointed out by Guyton et al. (1971), leaders of every related branch of science are agreed that there is instead a thin layer of gel, or a gelatinous matrix with minute interstices. These may be filled with ordinary liquid but do not intercommunicate. *It is to this liquid that we have restricted the old name 'interstitial fluid', and it is pressure within the interstices which we mean by the expression 'interstitial-fluid pressure'.* The gelatinous matrix would be permeable to molecules, but would not pass liquids in bulk.

A gel is a colloidal system in which particles of solid are dispersed in a liquid in a special way. Thus a colloid is a physical state rather than a category of substances. Indeed, most materials can be induced to adopt a colloidal state in the right circumstances. Physically a gel is an elastically deformable semi-solid, like a jelly. It can transmit a force to a limited extent, though rather less strictly unidirectionally than a solid can, nor can it flow like a liquid. Nor can it conduct ordinary equal-in-all-directions fluid pressure like a liquid. A gel has a capacity to imbibe water, but any such tendency in the interstitial compartment is opposed by the osmotic pressure of the plasma, drawing water into the capillaries.

When a cube of gel is immersed in water, the rate at which the water is imbibed is extremely slow. This rate is presumably a function of the area of the interface between gel and water. The time taken for the two to become one structure would depend upon the relation between the surface area and the volume of the gel. But the area of the surfaces of all the capillaries permeating a cube of tissue would be unimaginably vast compared with the area of the surface of a similarly-sized cube of gel. There seems to be no doubt that a substantial proportion of all the fluid that reaches the capillaries in the plasma, diffuses through their walls and back again during its transit through the tissues. It might have been expected that at any time a great deal of free fluid would be outside the vessels. Yet the tissues do not weep fluid when cut.

Could it be that as fluid escapes from the capillaries it immediately becomes part of the gel structure by a sort of instantaneous imbibition, so never appearing as free fluid except in the presence of pitting oedema? Oedema would then represent a sort of 'overflowing' of saturated gel.

Interstitial-fluid pressure

For many years interstitial-fluid pressure has been felt to be 'obviously' positive to atmospheric pressure. Popular argument ran thus. Skin being flexible must transmit atmospheric pressure. Also skin being demonstrably elastic, it must surely compress everything beneath it. Interstitial fluid must, therefore, be at atmospheric pressure plus something attributable to cutaneous elasticity. This argument would have been sound enough if skin had indeed floated on ordinary liquid, transmitting pressure in all directions. Instead if there is any liquid beneath normal skin it is certainly compartmentalised, or occupies the discrete interstices of a gelatinous matrix. Such pressure effects as would result from cutaneous tension would therefore be very strictly localized.

Moreover, elastic tension in the skin can exert pressure beneath it only where the skin is convex. Where the skin is flat its elasticity can have no effect on interstitial-fluid pressure. Where it follows a large hollow like the axilla, its elastic fibres are fully relaxed; and where there is no tension there is also no pressure effect. Where the skin conforms to small hollows like those between the knuckles, its elasticity must have a negative effect. If interstitial-fluid pressure were indeed positive one would expect these small hollows to fill with fluid, if nowhere else.

Beneath the skin there are countless coiled fibres of elastin, collagen, hyaluronic acid, etc., many or all of which are elastically compressible, like minute coil springs. According to the concept being described, these are surrounded by liquid at sub-atmospheric pressure. Accordingly the skin is sucked against these structures, or pushed against them by atmospheric pressure. Leaving aside such local effects as a subject's own weight pressing on the skin of the feet, or the weight of his clothes, the total pressure on the skin is atmospheric pressure. Wherever the skin is flat, this is equal to the pressure exerted against the structures that support the skin. But if any at all of this pressure is conducted through the fibres as what Ġuyton has called 'solid pressure', then the pressure in the interstitial fluid has to be sub-atmospheric.

Except by being sucked on, how else could the skin be made to conform to such hollows as that beneath the jaw? The explanation usually given is that it is held on by fibres or by a sort of glue. Years ago a popular method of treating dehydration in infants was by introducing a quantity of saline into the axillae. It used to be put straight in all together. Nevertheless, it used to go in very easily; and there was no evidence of dimpling, such as one might have expected. Moreover, it all used to disappear in an hour or two, which did not seem consistent with the notion of positive pressure beneath the skin.

We have heard protagonists of the notion of positive pressure beneath the skin, liken the fit of the skin to that of a rubber glove. In the main the rubber glove does fit as closely as the skin; but there is an important difference. This is in the fit between the knuckles and in the middle of the palm. These are the only parts of the hand that are concave, and here a rubber glove does not fit closely. Instead it bridges elastically from knuckle tip to knuckle tip, and across the centre of the palm.

At one time surgeons used to put on their sterile gloves under water. The excess water used to be allowed to drain out of the cuff, and as it did so, the glove used to be sucked everywhere against the hand. There were no fluid-containing spaces between the knuckles. But the potential space between the hand and the glove here was at subatmospheric pressure, like the potential space between the two layers of the pleura. This can be demonstrated thus. A surgical glove is put on under water in this way. The rubber between the knuckles is then nicked with scissors. Immediately a little air rushes in, and the rubber bridges elastically from knuckle to knuckle, exactly as in the glove put on in air.

As to the forces that maintain this subatmospheric level of pressure in the interstitial compartment, they are two. One is the sucking action of the initial lymphatics (as explained in the next chapter); the other is the net osmotic pressure of plasma drawing water and crystalloids through the capillary wall. Present estimates of the latter come to 18 mm Hg. (See Appendix no. 5.)

The measurement of interstitial-fluid pressure

Many attempts have been made to measure interstitial-fluid pressure directly. Most of even comparatively recent attempts involved injecting a tiny bead of liquid into the tissues, and trying to measure the pressure in the bead. But even the smallest of the beads would have been enormous compared with the imagined size of the interstices of the gel matrix, and been bound to distend such an interstice. A false positive record of pressure would therefore be expected. Guyton, who has been doing original and imaginative work in this field for many years, introduced a novel method of measuring interstitial-fluid pressure (Guyton, 1963). He implanted a small many-perforated capsule into the tissues. It soon became lined with tissue, and then filled with fluid, very like plasma, but with a protein content only about half as great. This fluid appeared to be in equilibrium with the interstitial fluid of the area in respect to both chemical and such physical characteristics as pressure. All who have tried the method have consistently recorded subatmospheric pressures in nearly every case. These have averaged 6 mm Hg beneath atmospheric pressure under the skin.

The chemical composition of the interstitial material

No one has ever isolated for certain a sample of what occupies the interstitial compartment, or even the mobile liquid part of it, though evidence is accumulating that the liquid part is indeed what fills Guyton's capsules. The mobile part, which we hold the old name 'interstitial fluid' should come to mean, appears to be capillary transudate. That is: it is the same as plasma in respect to water and crystalloids, and contains the same proteins at lower concentration, probably half as much. The protein content of lymph varies from place to place and from time to time, and probably that of interstitial fluid does as well accordingly.

The more permanent part of the material between the cells contains about 1 per cent of the muco-polysaccharide hyaluronic acid, said to be present as closely coiled fibrillae. There are also fibrils of collagen, and elastin. These materials help to give the matrix as a whole the physical characteristics described.

Formation and disposal at heart level

As has been explained, the material that occupies the interstitial compartment is certainly not ordinary liquid, though it is possible that the part of it that fills the imagined interstices of a gel matrix, may justly be so called. Much would depend on the size of these interstices, for the word 'liquid' is meaningless at the level of individual molecules. The state of liquidity arises from the pattern of arrangement of a number of molecules. Perhaps we may stretch the point, and refer to a 'potentially liquid' part of interstitial material. Anyway, only this part is concerned in constant exchange, or formation and disposal. A small amount of protein is involved, and will be considered in the chapter on lymph and the lymphatic system. Here we will consider only the water and crystalloids.

Diffusion is the result of rapid molecular movements and requires no gross physical force, or pressure difference. However, a difference of pressure on the two sides of a permeable membrane can determine that fluid *transfer* in one direction shall exceed that in the other.

Consequently, for diffusion to be directionally balanced it is necessary that pressures shall also be balanced, or diffusion in one direction will exceed that in the other until they become so. In exchanges between the blood and the interstitial compartment, four pressures are relevant, and may be grouped as two pairs, according to whether they encourage net outward diffusion (or extravasation) or net inward diffusion (or absorption), thus:

Pressure favouring extravasation:
    Intracapillary blood pressure;
    Osmotic pressure of peri-capillary material.
Pressures favouring reabsorption:
    Interstitial-fluid pressure;
    Osmotic pressure of plasma in relation to capillary walls.

At the arterial ends of capillaries with open precapillary sphincters, there is a good preponderance of transmural hydraulic pressure over net osmotic pressure. Extravasation must, therefore, occur there. At the speed at which such fluid transfer is now appreciated to take place, the pressures must come very quickly into equilibrium, for three different factors are exerting their influences simultaneously. Firstly, loss of water is causing the concentration of proteins in the plasma and their osmotic pressure to rise. Secondly, dilution of proteins in interstitial fluid is causing the osmotic pressure just outside the capillaries to fall. Thirdly, as the blood progresses along the capillary loop, its hydraulic pressure falls progressively. As the pairs of pressures approach equilibrium extravasation slows, finally stopping altogether, and then giving way to reabsorption. From here on there is no reason why the pressures should ever come out of balance again. In fact reabsorption may be relied upon exactly to keep pace with continuing fall of the hydraulic pressure of the blood and its net osmotic pressure.

(Pappenheimer (1953) emphasized that this kind of admittedly much simplified picture of fluid exchanges across capillary walls was apt to lead to misapprehension of its true nature. It could certainly lead to substantial error if applied to more refined calculations of the relation of pore size and numbers to fluid transfer rates. Pappenheimer pointed out that the fluid transfers through permeable membranes were of two different kinds, obeying different laws as to rate. Diffusion is the result of extremely rapid movements of individual molecules. Hydrodynamic flow, as Pappenheimer called it, occurs in response to a pressure difference (hydraulic or osmotic) and is essentially concerned with a

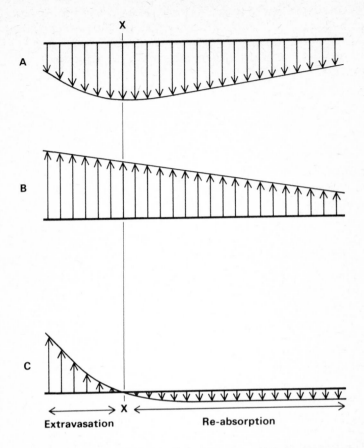

Fig. 11. *Imaginary graphs showing changes in size and direction of, A, net osmotic pressure between blood and interstitial material; B, transmural hydraulic pressure; and, C, net diffusion of water and crystalloids, during passage of the blood along a capillary loop (from left to right in the illustrations). X is the point of equality between osmotic and hydraulic pressure, when extravasation gives way to re-absorption.*

mass of molecules. Such bulk movement of fluid in obedience, for instance, to a law governing laminar flow through a tube-like pore could, of course, be expressed as a change in the average directional velocity of all the molecules of which the mass of fluid is composed; but they are not the same molecules as diffuse through a permeable membrane when they happen to strike it in the right place at the right minimum velocity. Whereas diffusion rate is directly related to total pore area, bulk flow is much more affected by individual pore sizes than by total pore numbers. In the formation or absorption of oedema it is bulk or hydrostatic flow that is important, while in the exchange of materials between blood and tissues, diffusion is many times more important.)

The fact that protein concentration in the plasma always remains well above that in the interstitial fluid, means that there is always net osmotic pressure drawing fluids into the capillaries, and that net hydraulic pressure to balance this will be maintained. In fact interstitial-fluid pressure is always held at a subatmospheric level, and the blood vessels are kept distended against their elastic walls at what has been called the 'basic pressure' of the blood. (See Appendix no. 2.)

Formation and disposal in dependent tissues

In dependent tissues the hydraulic pressure of the blood is greatly increased, for gravitational reasons, and extravasation at the arterial ends of open capillaries is even more assured. But reabsorption at their venous ends or throughout capillaries with closed precapillary sphincters, cannot be explained on the basis of currently accepted theory. Since Starling it has been thought that only plasma proteins are almost unable to pass through the walls of the capillaries, and therefore exert osmotic pressure. But everywhere in the capillaries of the lower limb of a standing man, the transmural hydraulic pressure of the blood greatly exceeds the net osmotic pressure of the proteins. It was suggested by Aukland (1973) that all the body had to do to compensate for a rise in venous (and capillary) pressure, was increase the relative area available for reabsorption, by increasing the proportion of closed precapillary sphincters. Such a mechanism might well operate for very modest elevations of venous pressure; but it could certainly not work in the feet of a standing man where the capillary blood pressure has risen 80 or 90 mm Hg; for here there is no area of reabsorption (on current theory) to enlarge.

One of us has suggested a way in which the so-called 'Starling Hypothesis' could be modified to adapt it to dependent tissues. This is that dependent capillaries become *less* permeable to some other larger-moleculed materials, as well as the proteins. These materials would then also exert their characteristic osmotic pressures. In this way it would be quite easy for net osmotic pressure to be made to match the increased hydraulic pressures in the feet on standing. If this hypothesis were true, certain materials present equally in plasma and interstitial fluid at heart level, would not be found, or be found less plentifully in interstitial fluid recovered from the feet. Comparison of the freezing points of the contents of Guyton capsules implanted in a foot and in the neck of a horse, are planned. It would be interesting to compare fluid samples from a foot and the scalp of a giraffe. We see no prospect of borrowing a giraffe in Britain, but perhaps one of our overseas colleagues will be better placed.

CHAPTER 6

Lymph and the Lymphatic System

THE NATURE AND SOURCE OF LYMPH

Most of the molecules of water and crystalloids of the plasma diffuse back and forth through the walls of the capillaries during the plasma's transit along these vessels, many of these molecules more than once. The capillaries are far less permeable to proteins, though a little does manage to escape. Some of this must diffuse back again, mostly that which never gets far from the capillaries; but the *transfer* of protein is not directionally balanced, on account of the adverse concentration gradient. There is net outward transfer of a few thousandths of the protein reaching the capillaries. All of this, plus the water in which it is dissolved after extravasation, plus any other solutes in the same water, finds its way into the lymphatic system. The lymph could be said to equal what has been extravasated from the capillaries, plus water and other metabolites diffused through the walls of the cells, minus what is absorbed back into the blood.

Accordingly, it has been assumed that because this is so it must be factors which affect extravasation or reabsorption that determine the rate of formation of lymph. Our own view is that this is put the wrong way round, and that it is the amount extravasated minus the amount that has been used as lymph that determines the quantity of fluids available for reabsorption. For, since fluids do not ordinarily accumulate in the tissues it would seem evident that the **whole** of what is not used to make lymph is reabsorbed, and that the volume of what becomes lymph is altogether independent of the quantities extravasated or reabsorbed.

The volume of lymph flowing in a limb varies a great deal with exercise, and so does the blood flow. Indeed, the two might have been guessed to be connected. But when the limb is held quite still lymph flow is reduced to zero, though blood flow is not. Also lymph flow is substantially increased by massage, while blood flow is not significantly affected. However, both exercise and massage activate the pumping mechanism of lymph (described shortly). This suggests that the rate of flow of lymph is much more influenced by its transport mechanism than by its rate of production. Indeed, we would question whether there is any such thing as a rate of production of lymph. Rather would we suggest that there is always ample fluid in the interstitial compartment, or the interstices of its gel matrix, to keep the lymphatics filled, whatever the rate of its transport along the lymph vessels, *and* leave plenty over for reabsorption. *For lymph flow is never more than a tiny fraction of the total quantity of fluids extravasated.*

According to our theory failure of lymph transport would never directly cause accumulation of water, for all that was not carried away in the lymphatics would simply be reabsorbed into the blood capillaries instead. Only proteins would accumulate. Normally the same things that promote increased extravasation of proteins also cause increased flow of lymph. Exceptions are damage to capillary walls, which does cause local accumulation of proteins, and massage. The latter encourages the flow of lymph without affecting the flow of protein.

The function of the lymph is to dispose of particles and effete or foreign cells that have gained access to the interstitial compartment, and to get rid of any excess of larger molecules unable to re-enter the capillaries and be carried away in the blood.

THE STRUCTURE OF LYMPHATICS AND THE FLOW OF LYMPH

The lymphatic system is not, as used to be thought, in full continuity with the interstitial compartment or with the serous cavities. With the coming of the electron microscope it has also become evident that the name 'lymphatic capillary' is quite unsuitable for the highly specialized structures at the beginning of the system. Indeed, it would better describe the smallest collecting channels, though best of all would be to discard the old name altogether to emphasize that the lymphatic system is not, like the vascular system, one with outgoing and ingoing vessels joined together by a capillary bed. It would also end all confusion with blood capillaries. A good name for these little structures at the beginning of the system is 'initial lymphatics', for they are larger than the earliest collecting vessels that follow them.

The initial lymphatics are blind ended and club-shaped (Fig. 12). Some are as much as 40 or 50μ in diameter. Their walls are very thin, consisting of a single layer of flattened endothelial cells with little or no basement membrane. The cells are not simply fitted together edge to

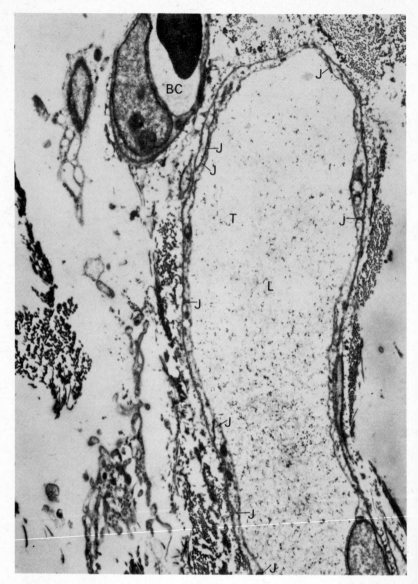

Fig. 12. Microphotograph of a single initial lymphatic vessel, × 7,000 (mouse). From Casley-Smith, J. R. (1970).

edge, but have irregular, sloping edges which overlap those of adjacent cells (Fig. 13A). They may be joined together only here and there, having a distinct, though often tortuous channel between them. These almost certainly open into the interstices of the gel matrix of the interstitial compartment. The initial lymphatics are less obviously supported by surrounding connective tissue than are blood capillaries, though an occasional fibril-like projection from the wall of an initial lymphatic appears to join it to a connective-tissue element.

(In the presence of oedema and raised interstitial-fluid pressure it might be thought that the initial lymphatics would become crushed, the flow of lymph diminished or halted and a vicious circle established, so that oedema, once started, would always become progressive. However, this does not in fact happen, and there are three reasons. First, it seems that each initial lymphatic must be partly or wholly within a minute cavity or interstice of the gel matrix of the interstitial compartment. The fibrils (say x of them), traverse this cavity to connective tissue in a far wall (see Fig. 13B). A rise of interstitial fluid pressure which tended to distend the cavity, would also tend to compress the initial lymphatic. Thus there would be exerted on each fibril an outward mean tension proportional to $R^3\pi/x$ and an inward tension proportional to $r^3\pi/x$, where R is the radius of a notionally spherical cavity and r is the radius of a notionally spherical initial lymphatic. The outward tension is the greater by a factor of $(R/r)^3$. Accordingly tension in the fibrils would in fact hold the initial lymphatic open.

Secondly, there is every reason to suppose that there is no hindrance to the entry of the initial lymphatics by all molecules. Therefore pressure within the initial lymphatic could not be less than outside it. Thus there is no fluid pressure difference to oppose the tension in the fibrils. Thirdly, it has been shown experimentally by Guyton et al. (1971) that there is a remarkable degree of tissue compliance to oedema. Interstitial-fluid pressure does not in fact rise significantly above atmospheric pressure before considerable oedema has occurred or been induced.)

The other function of the fibrils is to compel the walls of the initial lymphatics to follow all the little fortuitous movements that are occurring all the time in any living tissue. Some of these are associated with respiration; for little muscular adjustments to balance must be occurring all over the body of a standing creature; some result from more specific, local activity of skeletal or plain muscle; some are caused by arterial pulsation; others may even be Brownian movement.

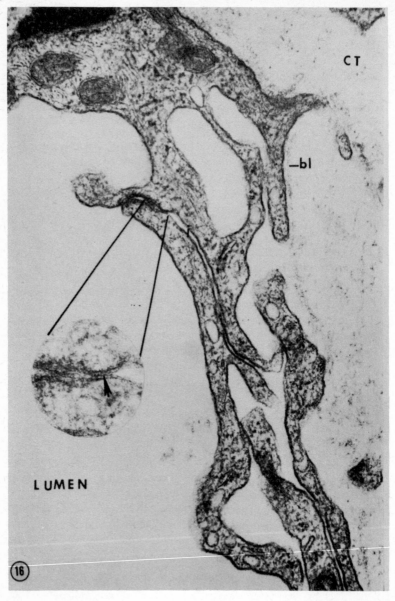

Fig. 13. A. Micrograph of part of the wall of an initial lymphatic × 69,000,
showing inter-cellular cannaliculi. At this magnification an
erythrocyte would be over 30 cm (a foot) broad. A tiny particle
appears to be passing along one cannaliculus.
Inset: this area is shown × 187,000.

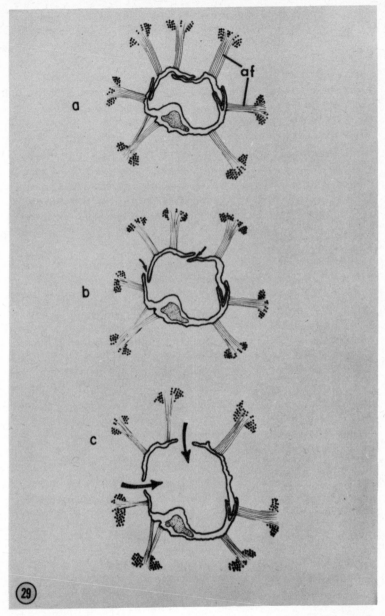

B. *Drawing to show how distension of the lymphatic will cause the overlapping edges of the cells to slide over one another, and finally to part and open up relatively large pores.*
Both figs. from Leak (1970).

Lymphatic vessels are closely valved right down to the junctions of the smallest collecting channels with initial lymphatics, the valves directing flow away from the periphery. Any little change of pressure relationship that tends to flatten an initial lymphatic also tends to close the intercellular cannaliculi, like a row of flap valves; while any movement that pulls the walls apart, also tends to open the channels. Thus the initial lymphatics would act like millions of ultra-microscopic enema syringes, each being repeatedly compressed and released. Each compression would, because of the arrangement of the valves, cause the initial lymphatic to force its contents into the related collecting vessel, while each relaxation would allow the initial lymphatic to fill passively with interstitial fluid at interstitial-fluid pressure. For reasons that were given in the last chapter we are satisfied that this is subatmospheric. Compression of the smallest of the collecting channels would work the same way, squeezing lymph from segment to segment, always proximally.

The larger lymph vessels, though still translucent, have a well-developed basement membrane, and a little circular and oblique muscle in their walls, into which amylenated nerve fibres may be traced. With the aid of their valves these channels are evidently capable of driving along their contents independently. The largest vessels have a trace of adventitia with vasa vasorum, as well as muscle, and are just visible to the naked eye. On account of their valves they have a closely beaded appearance. Those on the dorsum of the foot are about 0·3 mm across when distended, and have valves every 1·5 to 2·0 mm. In the thigh they are about the same size, but have valves only every 4 to 6 mm. The transport of lymph is also assisted by the major accessory venous pumps, and by the fact that many arteries share an inelastic muscle sheath with lymph vessels as well as with veins.

A system which moves its contents consecutively from one inter-valve segment to another, and never as a continuous column with all its valves open simultaneously, is not subject to more than insignificant hydrostatic effects. This is indeed what is observed when lymph pressures are measured at different levels in a standing subject. The physics of lymph transport is, therefore, different from that of blood in that it omits the syphon or 'U'-tube principle employed in the cardiovascular system, in that it moves the lymph from an area of low pressure to one of higher pressure, and in that it lacks a main, centralized pump. Instead, the whole system consists of a continuous row of tiny pumps, each stepping up the pressure a little more. Thus from one end of the system to the other, the pressure gradually gets higher, instead of gradually falling as it does in the cardiovascular system.

Years ago many people thought that there was a continuous gradient of pressure all the way from the tissue spaces to the great veins. However, one of us, with his colleagues made precise measurements of pressures in lymphatics of standing dogs. They showed that the pressures at the groin were always higher than those at the pad, and always higher in the thoracic duct than at the groin. Pressure in the great veins where the lymph duct terminated, was lower than at the end of the thoracic lymph duct, except at the end of expiration, when the valves at the end of the lymph ducts closed to prevent reflux of blood into the lymphatics (Calnan, Pflug, Reis, and Taylor, 1970). The orientation of the valves, as in the veins, makes it clear that, at least some of the time, it is a retrograde pressure gradient that has to be resisted.

The distribution of lymphatics varies a good deal as between one tissue and another. In the skin they are at least as dense as the blood capillaries, and they are rich in periosteum and fibrous planes. They are absent from bone marrow and in muscle are found only in fascia. Where they are plentiful lymphatics intercommunicate freely with others of similar size, and in some areas they form dense plexuses. Microscopically lymphatics in section are characteristically irregular. This would largely account for their very great distensibility.

Microscopic structure of lymph nodes

All lymph from tissues of the leg somewhere passes through a lymph node. One function of these is to filter off material not wanted back into the blood. The other is the formation and maturation of lymphocytes.

The lymph nodes form part of the reticulo-endothelial system. Each has a fibrous capsule from which trabeculae pass rather less than half way towards the depression of the hilum. Corresponding to this depth, the nodes are divided into outer cortex and inner medulla. The cortex contains the germinal centres, packed with developing lymphocytes. At their inner ends the trabeculae break up to form a fibrous mesh lined with branching, highly phagocytic reticulum cells.

Lymph enters the node by afferent vessels which join its periphery. After ramifying in the capsule, these open into the sinus-like lymph channel beneath its capsule. This everywhere separates the capsule from the cortex, and follows the trabeculae to the medulla, where it permeates its meshwork. The lymph is then gathered into efferent vessels which leave the hilum of the node. The hilum also receives an artery and vein, both of unexpectedly large size, and nerve fibres. These are mostly distributed to muscle in the capsule and trabeculae.

While lymph is in transit through nodes, particles of foreign matter, bacteria and cells, including malignant cells and some effete red cells, are ingested by the phagocytic reticulum cells, and mature lymphocytes are added. We have seen evidence of regenerated lymph vessels bypassing inguinal nodes which had been destroyed by radiotherapy.

The composition of lymph

The old, recently-discarded idea that lymph and interstitial fluid were the same thing, is now appreciated to be not so wrong after all. When two fluids are separated by a semipermeable membrane, persisting difference between them is dependent upon the permeability of the membrane. That is, upon the sizes of the apertures in the membrane in relation to the sizes of molecules and other particles in contact with it. In the case of interstitial fluid and lymph, the relevant membrane is the walls of the initial lymphatics. But these probably pass protein very freely. Indeed, bacteria, malignant cells, even particles of Indian ink appear to pass into the lymphatic system without difficulty.

So far as crystalloids and water are concerned, lymph and plasma are nearly identical, and it may be judged that liquid of the interstitial compartment is so as well. Only in respect to proteins do plasma and the mobile part of interstitial fluid differ, for blood capillaries are only very slightly permeable to these. In the case of lymph, fluid flow is entirely from interstitial compartment to lymphatics. Any hindrance to passage of proteins could result only in a higher concentration in interstitial fluid than in lymph. It seems to most workers in the field altogether more probable that proteins enter the lymphatics without any hindrance at all, and that in respect to protein concentration as well, lymph and interstitial fluid in the limbs, are the same (Yoffey and Courtice, 1970).

The actual protein concentration in lymph varies from time to time and place to place. At any particular time and place it must depend on the relationship between the rate of net outward diffusion of protein and the rate of volume flow of lymph from the same area in the same time. If products of metabolism and materials lost into the cells were neglected, the protein extravasated represented $x/1,000$ of the protein reaching the capillaries in the plasma in a certain area and time, and the lymph flow was $y/1,000$ of the blood flow in the same area and time, the concentration of protein in the lymph would average x/y of its concentration in the plasma. The whole of the protein of lymph is returned to the blood via the thoracic and other main lymph ducts, like other substances in solution. But particles and cells that have also entered the lymph in the tissues, are abstracted in the lymph nodes. At the same time lymphocytes are added.

PART II

Diseases.
Their Causes, Effects
and
Investigation

PREFACE TO PART II

General Concept of Major Venous Disease

Our observations on the anatomy of the venous system of the leg, and our whole concept of the pathogenesis of major venous disease, are so different from those currently taught, that we shall begin this part of our book with a general exposition of them. Views about less advanced venous disorder, and about lymphatic disease are either already various, or in accordance with our own ideas, and we shall deal with each as we come to it.

Anatomy

According to present teaching, the veins of the leg are divided into two systems by the fascia lata. The whole of the blood from the superficial system drains into the deep via the two saphenous veins, or via a limited number of very small veins called 'perforators'. All of these are guarded by valves directing flow exclusively from superficial to deep. In recent years, much of the pathology associated with venous disease has been blamed on incompetence of valves in these little veins.

This description of venous anatomy in the leg, has seemed to us inconsistent with clinical observation and with the established laws of fluid mechanics. Moreover, it has proved wrong on more exhaustive investigation. Firstly, it has been universal experience that when both saphenous veins have been stripped out, and all visible perforators tied, the superficial system has continued to drain perfectly satisfactorily. The reason for this became clear when we made this investigation. The veins of amputated legs were injected with Microfil, a material capable of entering the smallest vessels. The tissues were then examined microscopically. It was found that only the medium and larger veins were divided into two systems. There was no sign of any such division in the smallest veins or in the microcirculation. It is our view, therefore, that the larger part of the blood passing from superficial tissues to the deep venous system does so via the *microcirculation*.

We have also observed that many perforators are valveless, while a few others have valves turned in the opposite direction. We would also recall that applying Poiseuille's equation to expected flow in the perforators has this result. Even if the cross-sectional areas of all the perforators were to add up to the same total as that of the two saphenous veins, the same pressure head would be expected only to produce a few thousandths of the volume flow through perforators as through saphenous veins. At their *normal* size the perforators cannot have as important a role as has been suggested. This is not to deny the importance of ligating a perforator that has become dilated; nor that these little vessels are particularly apt to become dilated when a main deep vein is blocked.

Pathogenesis

Nearly all present notions about the way in which venous disease undermines the nutrition of the skin of parts of the leg are based on the 'venostatic concept'. According to this, the fundamental disorder is slowing of venous blood flow. It is well recognized that in major venous disease there is characteristically a substantial increase in overall venous capacity in the leg. This would indeed imply a diminished *velocity* of flow for the same *volume of flow* (see 'Flow', Chapter 1, no. 9). But according to the venostatic concept, loss of carrying capacity in deep veins has also reduced overall volume flow in the limb.

We do not dispute the importance of loss of carrying capacity in deep veins, on account of thrombosis, for example. But we recall that a deep thrombosis often takes many years to bring on evidence of loss of proper nutrition of certain areas of skin and subcutaneous tissue. Also ligature of the popliteal or the superficial femoral vein may be followed by no more than a little transitory oedema. It seems evident that it is not loss of a main deep vein that is directly responsible for trophic disturbance. We feel more inclined to lay the blame on the slowly developing dilatation of bypass channels. For it is an observable feature of veins all over the body that their blockage invariably leads to the dilatation of alternative channels. These are always available because of the very free communications that exist between veins, particularly the smallest ones.

As some of these become the easiest routes for the blood to take they become even more dilated; and it would be reasonable to suppose the dilatation to go right back to and include the arteriovenous capillaries. Thus the arterial blood finds easier, wider and more direct routes to the veins, instead of being divided between true capillaries as previously. This would explain why patients with advanced trophic changes benefit so much from often quite wide excisions of channels that have become dilated. It would also explain why blood in varicose veins is warmer and better oxygenated than that in normal veins.

To us, and indeed to a great many people, the word 'stasis' means diminished *velocity* of flow, and not necessarily diminished *volume* flow. While accepting that diminished velocity of flow may, and probably does, encourage thrombosis, we do not accept that it has anything to do with trophic changes. Poor nourishment of tissues would seem to us to imply inadequate blood supply; that is, diminished rate of volume flow *in the microcirculation*. We believe increased short circuiting of blood through dilated arterio-venous capillaries and venules to be the fundamental cause of trophic skin lesions of venous origin.

As to the fact that no obvious dilatation of arterio-venous capillaries has yet been reported, we would point out that even an amount of dilatation too small to be noticeable (especially when not deliberately looked for)—say 20 per cent, would be associated with some doubling of the blood flow for the same pressure-head. This would imply very considerable reduction of flow through true capillaries. Moreover, this is without even considering the possibility of undermining the contractility of the muscle of the arterio-venous capillaries, another possible effect of dilatation.

CHAPTER 7

Oedema

NATURE, ORIGIN, AND EFFECTS

The old idea of oedema as a simple excess of 'tissue fluid' is obviously inconsistent with the modern concept of an interstitial compartment filled with *gel*. However, the idea of oedema as consisting of **liquid** at least fits the clinical features of most **early** oedema and may be quite correct at this stage. What must be abandoned is the notion that oedema and interstitial 'fluid' are, physically or chemically, **necessarily the same.**

(It may be that in oedema there is liquid that has lifted the skin off the gel; or it may be that the first step in oedema formation is the conversion of the gel into a sol, which is then added to.)

Oedema is often described as the result of excess of extravasation over reabsorption by the capillaries. Such an imbalance would certainly lead to the accumulation of fluids in the tissues. Oedema would imply that a change had occurred in one or more of the four forces enumerated in Chapter 5. Either there had been an increase in capillary pressure, or in the osmotic pressure of the material in the interstitial compartment, or interstitial-fluid pressure had decreased, or the osmotic pressure of the plasma had decreased.

1. *Increased capillary pressure*

Capillary pressure increases and is an important contributory, if not the main, cause of oedema in heart failure and in venous obstruction. However, a far **larger** increase in capillary pressure occurs in the feet whenever the subject **simply stands up**.

(In capillaries with open pre-capillary sphincters this is immediate, for they are exposed to the full weight of the blood in the arteries, right to the top of the scalp. In capillaries with closed pre-capillary sphincters, the pressure rise is not absolutely immediate, for the blood in the larger veins cannot fall back into the capillaries on standing, owing to their valves. But a few capillaries always remain open; the venules are filled through these, until the pressure in the venules is high enough to lift the blood all the way to the heart. *All* capillaries are open to venules.)

Thus, within moments, the blood pressure in all capillaries in the feet, on standing, very greatly exceeds the osmotic pressure of plasma proteins. Why oedema does not promptly appear in the feet on standing is not yet known, though a hypothesis has been advanced in Chapter 5.

There would have been no problem if there had been continuous liquid in the interstitial compartment, but there are no hydrostatic effects in a gel, or in the compartmentalized liquid of the interstitial space.

Dependency does determine where an oedema of more general origin shall appear. Accordingly, the compensatory mechanism which protects tissues from the oedema effects of raised capillary pressure cannot be complete. In fact, pulmonary oedema does not develop until the pressure in the pulmonary vein has reached 25 or 30 mm Hg, and no overt oedema shows in a limb of which the venous pressure has been suddenly raised to 20 mm Hg (Aukland, 1973). **After these points it does.** Of the four pressures, the one most frequently disordered to the point of causing oedema is capillary pressure.

2. *Increased osmotic pressure of peri-capillary material*

The commonest cause of increase in osmotic pressure outside the capillaries leading to oedema, is escape into the interstitial compartment of organic materials from the blood, as a result of damage to capillary walls from trauma or of infection. Similar escape may be the cause of local swelling in such conditions as urticaria, believed to be an instance of disorder of capillary walls. **Probably all lymphoedema comes into this category**, owing to accumulation of proteins in the tissues because of a breakdown in the normal mechanism for their clearance (Fig. 14).

Lymphatic obstruction would be expected to result in an oedema of increasing protein concentration. Fluid can be obtained from the tissues only in the early stages of lymphatic oedema. Even so it is indeed usually of **high protein content** (Crockett, 1956). It would seem, therefore, that most or all lymphatic oedemas are promoted by the osmotic effect of retained protein rather than by a failure of fluid drainage.

3. *Reduced interstitial-fluid pressure*

The effect of reducing the interstitial-fluid pressure is seen when a rubber 'sucker' or a leech is applied to the skin and causes a little patch of oedema.

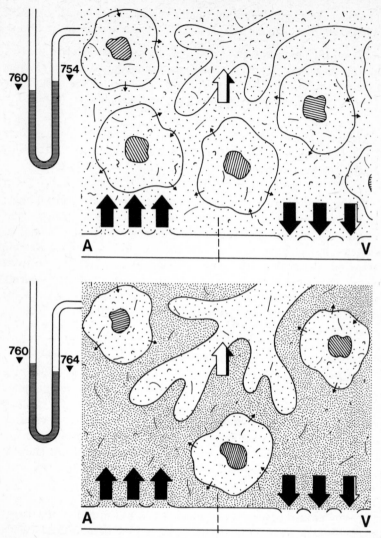

Fig. 14. To illustrate that fluid exchanges between blood and tissues are just as surely in balance in a static oedema as they are in normal tissue.

4. Diminished osmotic pressure of plasma

The oedema of diminished osmotic pressure of plasma is seen in nephrosis and in advanced starvation, with much reduced plasma protein level. Congenital absence of plasma protein is not associated with oedema, but it might be guessed that in this condition the capillary walls are impermeable to something else instead of protein, which therefore exerts osmotic pressure.

As would be expected, gravity has little effect on the location of oedemas of groups 2, 3, and 4.

In most patients with oedema, when first seen the oedema is in a relatively stationary state with the swelling neither getting rapidly worse, nor obviously absorbing. In these patients the four pressures must be just as certainly back in balance as they were before any oedema developed. This suggests that the **presence of oedema** so alters one or more of the other three pressures that it is able to compensate for the one that has been disordered, and bring the four back into equilibrium.

Oedema would not be expected to make any difference to capillary pressure nor to the osmotic pressure of plasma proteins. It was shown by Guyton et al. (1971) that in the presence of oedema interstitial-fluid pressure rose at least 6 mm Hg. Further discouragement to excess of extravasation over reabsorption would come from decrease in osmotic pressure of what surrounds the capillaries, and might be expected to result from accumulation of oedema. It is also likely to be much affected by the physical state of the material, as well as by the choice of chemical linkage, such as whether mucins and proteins are present in their separate identities or combined as muco-proteins.

The most important physical **effects** of oedema are upon interstitial-fluid pressure and its transmission. Guyton et al. (1971) showed that when one of their perforated capsules of water or saline was implanted in the tissues, its contents quickly came into equilibrium with tissue fluid, both in respect to chemical composition and in regard to physical characteristics, such as pressure. Under the skin the pressure averaged 6 mm Hg below atmospheric pressure. With the onset of oedema this pressure rapidly rose to zero, and remained at about that level until a great deal of oedema fluid had been accommodated. Thus a reserve of about 6 mm Hg of pressure existed before clinical oedema appeared. Another effect was on the conduction of pressure. If two capsules were implanted an inch apart, introducing liquid into one capsule to raise the pressure had no effect on the pressure in the other. As soon as oedema appeared or was induced, however, pressure **was** conducted from one capsule to the other, just as though only ordinary liquid lay between them (Fig. 15).

(Some have been puzzled why oedema does not cause blood capillaries and initial lymphatics to collapse. Blood capillaries are not threatened because the pressure inside a capillary is always higher than the pressure outside. Lymphatic vessels do not collapse for a reason described in Chapter 6.)

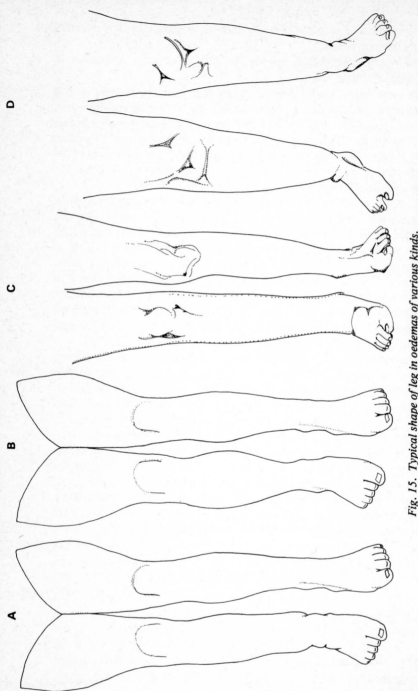

Fig. 15. Typical shape of leg in oedemas of various kinds.
A. Chronic venous insufficiency. The oedema is superficial.
B. Postphlebitic. The oedema is largely beneath the deep fascia.

CLASSIFICATION OF OEDEMA

Oedema has been classified by clinical features, by site, by believed causes, by age of onset, by expected duration and so on. But only in the light of modern methods of radiological investigation of both venous and lymphatic systems can oedema be divided satisfactorily. **Venous, lymphatic and non-vascular oedema may be recognized according to whether or not there is a demonstrable lymph vascular or blood vascular cause. While agreeing that most venous oedema comes and goes completely, and most lymphoedema is largely irreversible, we cannot accept that lymphoedema is synonymous with chronic oedema.** It may be true that oedema of lymphatic origin never completely disappears with recumbency, though most patients show noticeable improvement if elevation is maintained for several days. There are also cases of oedema of venous origin which largely lose their response to elevation, and we cannot accept that they should then be called 'lymphoedemas'.

CLINICAL FEATURES

Clinically oedema is defined as 'pitting' or 'solid'. By 'pitting' is meant swelling of the superficial tissues that can be displaced locally by pressure. If pressure with a finger tip is maintained over a bony surface for several seconds, when the finger is removed a distinct or even obvious pit remains for many minutes. Such oedema is evidently liquid, for gel cannot be altered in shape in this sort of way. A gel is deformable to a limited extent, but only elastically so. 'Solid' oedema cannot be pitted, though it must have started as a pitting oedema to have justified the name 'oedema' at all. It used to be assumed to have clotted. Oedema that has a high protein content tends to become solid much more rapidly than other oedema. Solid oedema is little affected by local compression or by elevation, while pitting oedema responds to either, particularly if of general origin such as in heart failure.

Another way of distinguishing oedema clinically is according to the tissue or depth of tissue involved. In the great majority of cases in which the name 'oedema' is used the liquid accumulates between the deep fascia and the skin. But there is a rare type of oedema in which the swelling is *in* the skin, and may be absent beneath it. This kind of oedema is mostly seen in certain cases of malignant disease and is known as **'peau d'orange'**. In this condition the lymphatics leading from the dermis proper have become blocked. The skin itself swells, and where the swelling has been prevented by tension on Cooper's ligaments, little pits like those in the skin of an orange, are seen. In severe obstruction of deep veins, fluid may accumulate beneath the deep fascia. This is characterized by change of shape of the leg (see Chapter 10. Deep Oedema).

The first thing to observe about oedema clinically is whether it is bilateral and confined to dependent areas, or whether it is a local and unilateral manifestation, or at least obviously different on the two sides. If the oedema is suspected of being of general origin one will need to observe whether there is dyspnoea or persisting tachycardia on moderate exertion, whether there is hypertension or evidence of chronic bronchitis, or whether there is protein in the urine.

When the oedema is apparently of local origin, one is interested in the family history, the duration, the variability and when this is present, the things that make the swelling worse. One will look for other evidence of venous or lymphatic disease, after eliminating any questions of local infection or trauma, not forgetting chronic traumatic lesions like certain ligamentous disorders, or diseases of joints, bursae, etc. Though one may prefer to find a single cause, one factor tending to promote oedema may facilitate another which might not have caused clinical oedema by itself.

INVESTIGATION

Radiological investigation involves much discomfort for the patient, and should not be undertaken lightly; but there are situations in which it is clearly called for. In cases of uncertain origin, at least one of the radiological investigations will be undertaken, and often both phlebography and lymphography. Phlebography is also necessary in the diagnosis and proper management of acute thrombosis. It is also called for before any kind of surgery in which deep veins are involved. Electrophoresis of plasma proteins is sometimes indicated; also electrocardiography, and of course urine analysis.

Phlebography

We do not recommend phlebography unless we are satisfied that it may give information that can help in the treatment of the patient. However, some clinicians believe in using it routinely even when no more than ordinary varicose veins are present, and no swelling. In such patients a suitable vein is sometimes visible through the skin of the foot. Percutaneous cannulation may then be performed. When the foot is swollen, however, there is no alternative to a cut-down technique. Moreover, we would not accept that the need for this should ever be considered a contraindication to phlebography, when one is really called for.

Phlebograms used to be made by injecting radio-opaque material and then making radiographic exposures at guessed intervals. The results were somewhat 'hit or miss'. Screening control was not possible on account of the large dosage of X-rays that would have been necessary. Now, with the aid of image intensification and closed-circuit television, there is no longer any problem. The operator may himself watch the material pass along the vessels and signal the radiologist when he wants an exposure. In fact, so much have results improved that it is now seldom justifiable to attempt phlebography unless an image intensifier and television screen are available in the radiology department.

Instruments and materials for phlebography

1. Three 20 ml syringes for Lipiodol or other contrast medium.
2. 5 ml syringe for local anaesthetic.
3. Gauge 22 hypodermic needles.
4. Scalpel handle with No. 15 blades.
5. Four curved mosquito artery forceps.
6. Two pairs of scissors.
7. Addison's dissecting forceps.
8. Two non-toothed dissecting forceps, as used by eye surgeons.
9. Small, light needle holder.
10. Small, curved cutting needles.
11. Gauge 16 to 18 polythene cannulas.*
12. 0000 plain catgut.
13. 0·5 per cent Lignocain *with* adrenalin.
14. Small swabs.
15. Smallest adhesive steristrip for fixing cannula.
16. Polymixin spray.
17. Small adhesive waterproof dressings.
18. At least 60 ml of Lipiodol for blood-vessel use.
19. Towel clips.

* These cannulas are made by Bard Ltd. They consist of a fine polythene tube mounted on a long, hollow needle. Both the needle and the cannula have shanks to fit a syringe.

Ascending phlebography

The radiologist will need to know just what it is hoped to demonstrate, in order that he may be able to co-operate, for phlebograms vary in the details of their planning, and are not the routine procedures they are often imagined to be by clinicians.

An 8 to 10 mm longitudinal incision is made under local anaesthesia

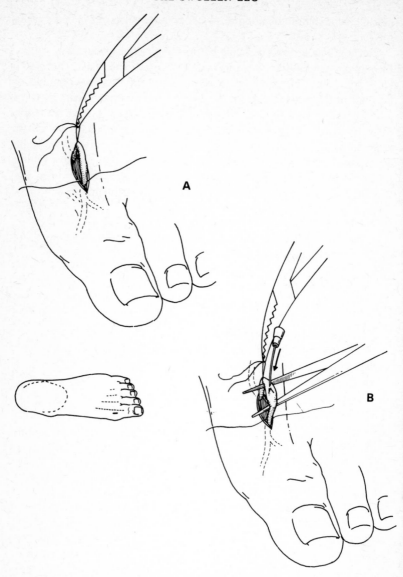

Fig. 16. A. The medial dorsal vein of the great toe is exposed over the first
              metatarsophalangeal joint. (This is often more than a cm on the
              foot side of the proximal end of the first interdigital cleft.) Inset, to
              show position of incision.
        B. The vein is dissected out and delivered by blunt dissection, and held
              for the introduction of the cannula, as shown.

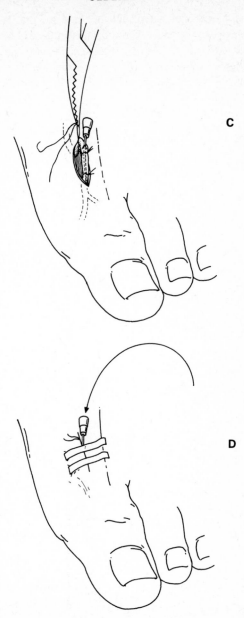

C

D

C. *The cannula is doubly tied into the vein.*
D. *The wound is closed and the tube attached to the cannula strapped to the skin.*

over the metatarso-phalangeal joint of the great toe, just to the medial side of the extensor tendon. The medial dorsal vein of the great toe is isolated and tied off at the proximal end of the incision with 0000 chromic catgut. The ends of this ligature are left long and are used to control the vein while it is cannulated (Fig. 17). (They may also be useful subsequently for recovery of the vein should the cannula slip out during nursing procedures.) The small polythene cannula is introduced directed distally (Fig. 16B), and tied in twice. (These ligatures must not crush the

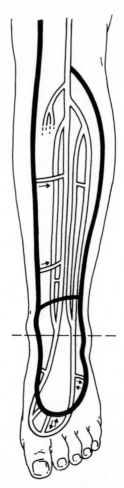

Fig. 17. *A venous tourniquet above the ankle compels all blood from the foot to enter the deep venous system, as will be seen by studying the above diagram.*

cannula.) A length of light rubber tubing is fixed around the leg above the ankle to act as a venous tourniquet. It should be no tighter than necessary to obstruct the superficial veins, and direct the contrast medium into the deep system. 30 to 50 ml of 45 per cent contrast is injected. After the procedure, it is a wise precaution to inject 5,000 U of heparin through the cannula.

After the films have been confirmed to be satisfactory the cannula is withdrawn, the vein tied with 0000 catgut and the skin wound closed. A firm crêpe bandage is applied for 24 to 48 hours.

This investigation should demonstrate:

1. Patency and any anatomical abnormality of the deep veins. The superficial veins will be shown instead of the deep if there is incompetence of a perforator above the tourniquet, or if the venous tourniquet is dispensed with.

2. Competence of perforating veins of both lower leg and thigh.

3. The rate of clearance of the whole system.

4. The function of the calf pump may be investigated by flexing and extending the ankle while injecting opaque medium. This is called 'dynamic phlebography'.

Descending phlebography

This method is occasionally used to demonstrate competence or otherwise of the valves of the deep veins and of the smaller perforators. (Competence of the valves at the mouths of the saphenous veins is easily demonstrated clinically.) The injection is most often made into the proximal end of the common femoral vein through a polythene catheter introduced by the Seldinger technique. Films are exposed before and during a Valsalva manœuvre to promote retrograde flow if the valves are incompetent. The catheter may then be pushed proximally and further injection and exposures made to demonstrate the state of the iliac veins.

Intraosseous phlebography

Injection of contrast medium may be made through special intraosseous cannulae into the calcaneous or into both malleoli, to visualize the veins of the lower leg. Particularly good pictures of deep veins are obtained. The femoral condyles are chosen for the thigh, and the great trochanters for the pelvic veins and vena cava. The procedure requires general anaesthesia, and subsequently there is pain at the site of injection, which may persist for several weeks. This can be largely eliminated by flushing out the area with 5,000 U of heparin, and leaving in 20 mg of hydrocortisone.

Complications of phlebography

Apart from infection of the wound, which is commoner than it should be, there are two potentially more serious complications. Fortunately both are rare, at least as clinically manifest conditions. One is hypersensitivity to the contrast medium, almost unknown with modern preparations. However, resuscitation apparatus should always be on hand, and someone present who knows how to use it. Indeed, this is something every nurse and doctor should be conversant with. The apparatus consists of a simple balloon rebreather and face mask, to facilitate forced inflation of the lungs with air. Oxygen is quite unnecessary and has no particular advantage over air. In an emergency, mouth-to-mouth respiration can save life.

The other complication is thrombosis induced by the injection. Thrombosis is very rarely large enough to cause signs or symptoms. However, in those who happened to be operated upon shortly after phlebography, we have observed small thrombi in no less than 30 per cent. This is why we have recommended that 5,000 units of heparin should be given after every phlebography.

Lymphography

Conventional lymphography, as still frequently done, was planned before it was appreciated that lymph drainage was normally strictly regional. In effect it was limited to the vessels of the medial superficial group, and missed those of the lateral superficial group, as well as the whole of the deep system. Most of the inguinal and pelvic nodes were reached, though there were a few that were not, for they receive all their lymph from the deep system. We have therefore worked out the following modified technique. The old watery solutions of dye had to be abandoned, for they used to leak into the tissues and spoil the pictures. It must be accepted, however, that the oily solutions now used may be less physiological, though they may be much better suited to the unphysiological rates of flow (and injection pressures) that have to be used.

Instruments and materials

These are almost the same as for phlebography (see this chapter). Superfluid Lipiodol (specially for lymphatics) is used instead of ordinary Lipiodol. There must also be some patent blue, and an extra, small syringe for it. Instead of the cannula for phlebography, one specially made for lymphography is used. It has a polythene shank to fit a syringe.

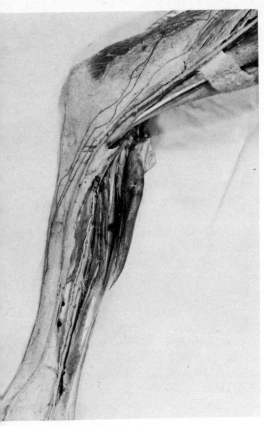
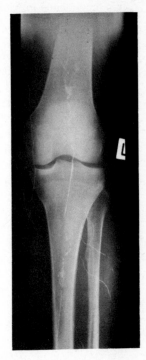

Fig. 18. A. An amputated leg after dissection of lymphatics.
      B. The lymphatics have been injected with Lipiodol and can be seen in
        the radiograph.

This is attached to about a metre of very fine polythene tube. At its other end this tube terminates as a tiny hollow needle.

Each big syringe is charged with 7 ml of Lipiodol, the limit for each leg.

Medial superficial system

0·3 ml of patent blue solution (anything from 2 to 10 per cent has been used with equal success) is mixed with 0·2 ml of 0·5 per cent Xylocaine. This is injected subcutaneously into the web space of the first interdigital cleft. In 10 to 15 minutes, if lymphatics are present, bluish streaks appear on the dorsum of the foot. Sometimes there are white streaks, presumably due to spasm of blood capillaries induced by the material injected. The blue streaks overlie lymphatic trunks, and the white streaks usually do so as well, though occasionally a white streak is found to overlie a small vein. In either case a lymph trunk is sought through a 5 mm longitudinal incision. This is made over a streak, choosing a blue one if there are both. This is done under local anaesthesia, for which we use about 2 ml of 0·5 per cent Xylocaine. Some have opposed the use of adrenalin as well, on the ground that it might promote spasm of the lymphatic trunk; though on the contrary, we urge its invariable use in order to achieve the bloodless field that we consider essential to successful lymphography.

If a trunk is found, at least 3 mm must be cleaned of adjacent tissue in order that the spiral shape of the lymphatic may be straightened out, so that it can be held in line with the cannula, to avoid puncture of the far wall. The special gauge 27 cannula is inserted and tied into the trunk with 0000 catgut, using a single knot so that it may be easily released in due course, with minimal danger of injury to this delicate structure. Into the cannula is injected 7 ml of Lipiodol (Ultrafluid), using a pressure of 6 lb. on the plunger of a 20 ml syringe.

In the presence of lymphatic oedema the streaks usually do not appear, and a suitable trunk must be sought blindly. The distal third of the dorsum of the foot is prepared for more extensive dissection. Under local anaesthesia with adrenalin a 1·5 to 2 cm incision is made over and in line with the extensor hallucis tendon. If no suitable trunk is found in the incision, further search is made under the skin on either side. If a trunk is found here, an incision directly over it will be necessary before more detailed dissection and cannulation are attempted. If still no lymphatic is found, a similar search is made of the **lateral** half of the dorsum of the foot. First another injection of dye will be necessary. This time it is made into the fourth interdigital cleft. If still no lymphatic is found, so-called 'aplasia' of the lymphatics of the *medial* region, and this region alone, may be judged to be present. The more experienced the operator the less often is the diagnosis of 'aplasia' made.

The lateral superficial system

The next step is investigation of the **superficial lateral** region. An injection, exactly as used previously, is put subcutaneously beneath the lateral malleolus (Fig. 19). Under local anaesthesia a 1 to 1·3 cm incision is made behind the lateral malleolus, over the short saphenous vein. The lateral superficial lymph trunk is most often medial and deep to the vein. The vein is held clear by tape and at least 3 mm of lymph trunk dissected free as described above, cannulated and injected. If no trunk is able to be

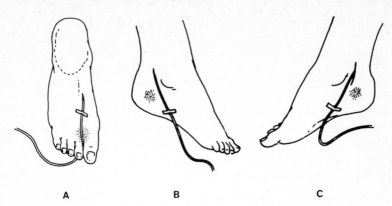

Fig. 19. A. The cannula inserted for medial superficial lymphography in the right foot.
B. Lateral superficial lymphography in the right foot.
C. Deep lymphography in the right foot.

found at this site either, the diagnosis of aplasia of the whole superficial lymph system may be deemed to have been established. The deep system is now investigated.

The deep system

The relevant trunk in the presence of lymphatic oedema lies at a depth of some 2 or 3 cm, and suitable retractors must be available. The technique of cannulation of a deep lymphatic trunk is difficult and involves precarious handling of the posterior tibial venae commitantes.

The area below and behind the medial malleolus is anaesthetized. The patent blue and Xylocaine is injected onto the outside of the periosteum of the calcaneous. A 2 to 2·5 cm curved incision is made over the posterior tibial vessels; the aponeurosis is opened, and the posterior tibial artery exposed, dissected free and taped, so that it can be held aside without injury. The posterior tibial lymphatic lymph trunk lies between the artery and its venae commitantes. This time 10 or 12 mm of lymphatic will be required, owing to the greater depth of the dissection. Dissection, cannulation, and injection proceed as described above.

In the course of 50 deep lymphographies we have not encountered a condition which we could have called 'hyperplasia'.

Complications

Hypersensitivity both to the Lipiodol and to the patent blue have been described, but we have not encountered either. Anaphilaxis should be dealt with as described under 'Complications of phlebography' in this chapter.

Rupture of a lymphatic trunk can occur if too high an injection pressure is used. It is necessary to remember that lymph flow is normally extremely slow, and to be very patient. Should the accident occur, the extravasated material is best evacuated through a small incision. It is too thick to be able to be aspirated.

Lung embolism can occur with use of a dangerously large dose of contrast medium. We have not experienced it with a total dose limited to 7 ml per leg, and at a plunger pressure on a 20 cc syringe not exceeding 6 lb. Our radiologists have given up taking check pulmonary radiographs.

CHAPTER 8

Varicose Veins

It has been estimated that in Europe and North America 20 per cent of women and 7 per cent of men have some disorder of the veins of the leg, of which far the commonest is varicose veins.

Healthy young people are not aware of their leg veins, nor are these visible. With advancing age the skin becomes thinner and less elastic, and the veins become wider and less contractile. In about a third of normal women and two-thirds of normal men over the age of thirty-five years, some of the larger veins do become visible under the skin, especially if the legs have undergone excessive strain. When they are particularly prominent, and when the name is appropriate, they are called 'athlete's veins', for it is in bicyclists and such that they are most apt to become conspicuous. The main trunks can become very large, but they retain a straight, normal course, and are symptomless.

Spider veins

Very small dermal veins also may become visible as bluish pencillings, either individually or as confluent groups, and are called 'spider veins'. These tiny vessels are permanently dilated, and are often said to have lost their tone. However, the larger a vessel becomes the greater the tension required in its muscle to overcome a given pressure within it. Every vessel must, therefore, have a sort of 'point of no return' which these little veins seem to have exceeded. They are especially inclined to appear quite early in pregnancy, before any mechanical effects can have arisen, and they are therefore judged to have been hormonally promoted. They cause no symptoms and have only cosmetic significance.

True varicose veins

True varicose veins are veins that have become visibly distended and tortuous. In places the walls are thinned by stretching, in others thickened by infiltration with fibrous tissue, together causing sacculation. The elastic fibres disappear, and later much of the muscle. The previous distinctness of the layers of collagen and muscle is lost. The sacculations

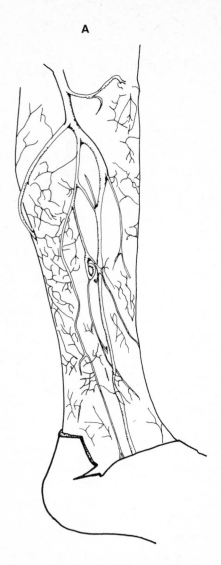

Fig. 20. To show the dense network of veins typical of varicose vein subjects and
the loss of normal hierarchy of superficial veins. Large, tortuous veins
appear where none were apparent at all previously.
A. Normal. B. Varicose veins.

B

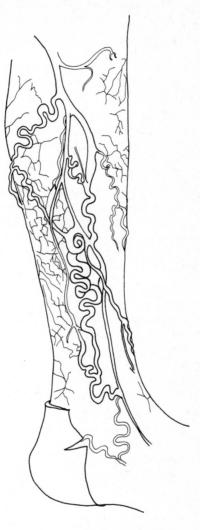

and general distension become rigid, hard, and fixed, and the tortuosities become matted together by fibrosis. There is also usually a demonstrable disorder of function, such as evidence of valvular incompetence (not always associated with obvious anatomical derangement) and even of retrograde blood flow (Fig. 20).

PATHOGENESIS AND CLASSIFICATION

Traditionally varicose veins were divided into 'primary' and 'secondary'. But the great majority of those that were thought to have had clear precipitating factors were found to be indistinguishable from ones held to be primary, either in their histological appearances, or in their clinical course. On the other hand, the somewhat different changes, with widespread dilatation of intradermal veins, that characterized some of the worst cases of deep venous obstruction, rarely followed exposure of a vein to blood at arterial pressure. In fact, when a vein is used to replace a diseased segment of artery, or an orthopaedic surgeon makes an artifical arterio-venous aneurysm to promote leg growth, the expected gross varicosity does not follow. Instead, the vein becomes 'arterialized'. Clinically the vein becomes much enlarged, but remains straight and regular. Microscopically there is great thickening of the wall, with marked muscle hypertrophy, but no lengthening and tortuosity.

There seem to be three distinct kinds of possible venous response to high venous blood pressure. It may well be the range into which the operative pressure falls that determines which kind of response shall occur. The highest range seems to promote such rapid thickening that lengthening does not have time to develop. There is also the fact that the longitudinal tension is always exactly half the circumferential tension, resulting from intraluminal pressure. The middle range causes all veins to become dilated, but conspicuously affects quite small intradermal veins. The lowest range takes longest to operate, and produces changes that are essentially patchy and regional. These are the changes in which a predisposing factor must most operate. For it is certainly not level of pressure that determines which veins in a leg shall first become varicose. Indeed, the presence of a venous disorder cannot make nearly so much difference to the pressure in a vein as can postural hydrostatic effects. A vein at the ankle will often have to cope with twice the level of pressure sustained at the groin. Yet it is often nearer the groin that an ordinary varicosity first appears.

It is ordinary varicose veins that are being described in this chapter, and we have adopted the view that in most, if not in all cases, more than one factor has been involved in aetiology. Accordingly we shall abandon the old names, 'primary' and 'secondary'. The rather different changes sometimes seen after severe deep thrombosis will be described in the chapter on the Postphlebitic Syndrome.

Of patients who get deep venous thrombosis, only a few of the worst later develop this special variety of widespread dilatation of small superficial veins. Far the commonest kind of venous disorder to come on after deep vein thrombosis is ordinary varicose veins, indistinguishable from ones that have appeared in a patient who has not had a deep thrombosis. Moreover, a patient who already has ordinary varicose veins is more apt to develop deep thrombosis than one whose superficial veins are normal.

At the same time, patients are not commonly met with who have one kind of venous abnormality in one part of a leg, and another kind elsewhere. It is more as though a balance for type of venous response having been struck for one set of circumstances in one particular patient, that balance applied for the whole patient, from then on. The extent of inborn defect would be an important factor in determining the type of response. It must be largely inborn defect also that determines that one particular vein shall become varicose, and another not.

The factors that give rise to fully-developed varicosity may be divided into two groups: (1) the primary cause that predisposes to the giving way of a particular valve, or to a particular segment of vein becoming varicose; and (2), those that are responsible for the invariably progressive worsening of the condition.

Primary factors

The first are essentially local in their effect, greatly varying in extent from vein to vein, or so it would seem. Like all morphological characteristics, these structural ones that predispose to varicosity are strongly hereditary. (There is even a tendency for varicosity to appear at the same site in offspring as in parents.) They seem to be present to some extent in most human beings, though not in other animals. Another factor operates early in pregnancy. Like the preponderance of female sex among varicose-vein subjects, this is assumed to be hormonal. Also, it has recently been reported that negroes seem to be racially immune while living in their natural environment. But when they live in cities and adopt local ways they have a similar incidence of varicose veins to that of their white neighbours. This has been attributed to absence of adequate roughage from 'civilized' diet (Burkitt, 1972).

Some people have argued that there are no such things as truly primary or idiopathic varicose veins, and that at least to some extent one

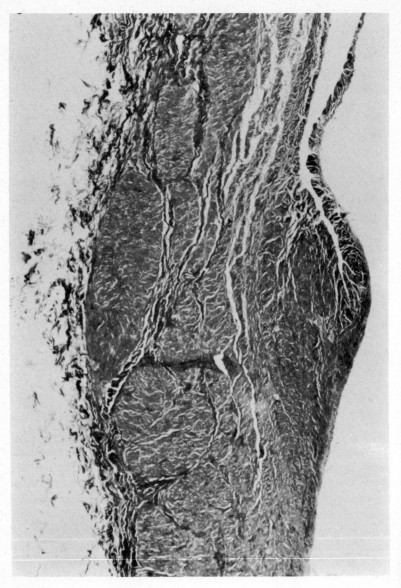

Fig. 21. A. Microscopic view of a section of a normal valve cusp. The lumen of the vein is to the right.

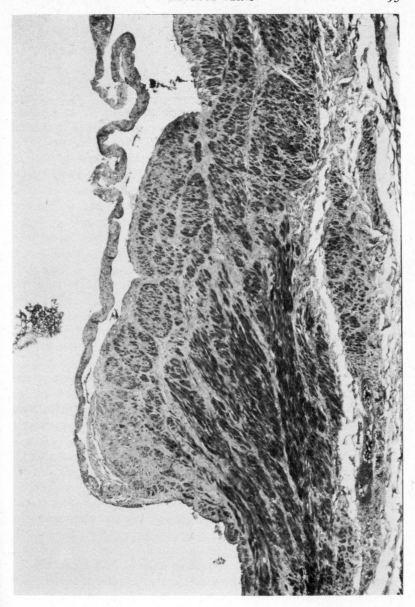

B. A valve involved in the varicose process. There is great hypertrophy of the muscle of the valve. The lumen of the vein is to the left.

of the factors in the second group must contribute in every case. Their argument is irrefutable if we are to include the high level of hydrostatic pressure that normally operates in the feet of a standing man; for varicose veins never appear in the arms.

Exactly what the hereditary defect consists in that predisposes to varicosity is not yet established. Some have felt an unsatisfactory proportion of collagen, elastin, and muscle elements to be an adequate explanation (Svejcar et al., 1961); others have suggested congenital absence of the valves (Basmajian, 1952; Lodin and Lindvall, 1961). Yet others have thought they saw evidence of complete disappearance of valves in radiographs, and have judged this to have been due to a congenital weakness (Dos Santos, 1948). We would add another vague suggestion (not very seriously) that there is a neurological malfunction with active opening of otherwise normal valves at wrong times.

An important paper by Piulachs and Vidal-Barraquer appeared in 1953. Unfortunately, it was very long and rather 'solid' reading, which may be why it did not continue to attract the attention it merited. It contained some excellent and original observations which, so far as we can ascertain have never been either contradicted or confirmed. Nor have alternative explanations been proposed. The most important of these observations was that radio-opaque material introduced into arteries took much less time to appear in veins in varicose-vein subjects than in normals. They also confirmed the observation, first made by Blalock (1929), that the O_2 saturation of blood from most varicose veins was *above* that of blood from corresponding contralateral normal veins (see Bibliography). We would guess our own observation of increased skin temperature over varicose veins to have the same explanation, whatever that finally turns out to be.

Piulachs and Vidal-Barraquer put forward the hypothesis that all varicose veins arose on a basis of congenital excess of small arterio-venous communications; an idea supported by Bassi (1956) and later by Haeger and Lindell (1966). Indeed, Piulachs and Vidal-Barraquer had dissected some out in varicose-vein subjects. They also postulated what they called 'starting agents', which caused the hitherto latent connections to open up. One of these they held to be trauma, for they had noticed that in their own series, varicosity seemed so often to have begun with an injury. Another they held to be warmth, for they considered the incidence of varicose veins to be higher in hot climates than in colder ones. As a third they mentioned pregnancy. They made no suggestion as to how their starting agents might operate.

Although we regard this as the best attempt so far made to explain observable facts about varicose veins, facts which have been so widely ignored, we cannot accept that Piulachs and Vidal-Barraquer hit on the right answer. They claimed that their arterio-venous communications were present to varying extents in everyone. There does not seem to have been any question of their having had in mind the arterio-venous capillaries described in Chapter 3; for these are universal, and could not very well have been more numerous in varicose-vein subjects than in other people. Larger arterio-venous connections do exist in certain parts of the body, but none have yet been described in the limbs.

However, it is arteriovenous capillaries which, along with their associated venules, we believe to become sufficiently dilated to be able to be dissected out in certain circumstances. We do not accept that they are ever present in abnormal numbers, varying instead only in the extent of their dilatation and the proportion dilated. Nor can we regard them as ever a primary cause of varicosity, since in our view, their dilatation is itself a secondary phenomenon and is due to their having become part of a preferred route for the blood.

Preferred routes

Blood from the capillaries has a number of alternative routes through veins. **Which route it chooses is not a matter of chance**. Indeed, radio-opaque material injected into a vein is seen always to take the same route. *The proportion of the blood which follows each of alternative routes is bound to be in the inverse ratio of their resistances*. The resistance of a vessel per unit length to the flow of plasma is in inverse proportion to (the radius of a vessel)[4]. Blood is not very different. Thus a small addition to the calibre of one route can cause it to be preferred to another by a surprisingly large factor. Moreover, for any given head of pressure in its contents, the circumferential tension in the walls of a vessel is proportional to its width. Accordingly, the more a vessel dilates, the larger the tension in its walls for the **same** head of pressure. The establishment of a preferred route is therefore something of a vicious circle. Everything is in favour of the development of clinically obvious pathological circuits.

We would accept that anything that physiologically promotes prolonged opening of arterio-venous capillaries could help to start a 'preferred route' for the blood.

Thus, according to our concept, the hereditary feature which predisposes a particular vein to become varicose is *local* weakness of the whole vein wall *in proportion to the pressure that it has to withstand there in the circumstances of that patient's life, and in proportion to the diameter of the vein at that point.*

Secondary factors

The second group of factors, those that both hasten the onset of varicose veins, and doom the condition always to pursue its inexorable downhill course, are more straightforward, and are these: (1) deep venous obstruction; (2) the giving way of key valves; (3) loss of the usual size relationship between superficial veins and the deep veins into which they drain; (4) loss of the normal hierarchy of superficial veins and the 'Laplacian advantage' that goes with it; and (5) occupational factors that lead to superficial veins being exposed to excessive pressure, or overlong exposure to pressures ordinarily encountered for only moments.

Normal veins often have to cope with moments of high pressure, but are usually quickly relieved by activation of one of the muscle pumps. Failure to use these pumps commonly precipitates varicosity. The effects of all these factors are best considered by following the course of venous drainage in the leg during walking.

Pressure changes in the leg veins during walking

A. Normal

As the calf muscles of a normal standing man contract, the pressure of the blood in the sinusoidal veins of the calf muscles and the superficial veins is about the same at the same levels. The muscle pump has not yet come into operation. If the man takes a step and the calf muscles contract, the sinusoidal veins within them are powerfully compressed. Provided all valves protecting superficial from deep veins are intact, and provided there is an adequate route for the blood via other deep veins, all the blood from the sinusoids is promptly squeezed into these, and on towards the heart. There is no reason or need for pressure in these deep veins to rise more than momentarily. There is, of course, a wave of high pressure which normal, well-supported deep veins and healthy valves can very well withstand. As soon as the calf muscles relax pressure in the sinusoids falls sharply by 50 per cent or more. Blood from superficial veins is able to pour into the now empty sinusoids. Pressure in the superficial veins therefore also falls.

This blood used to be thought all to go via so-called 'perforator veins', a limited number of small but visible veins, but our own belief is that much more of it goes by innumerable, microscopic veins.

B. After a deep vein thrombosis

If the main deep veins are partially or completely obstructed, however, a much longer-sustained rise of pressure occurs in the calf sinusoids after calf contraction before all the blood manages to get away. Obviously the effect will be commensurate with the extent of the block. The effect will also depend very much on the state of the valves in deep veins and on those protecting the superficial veins. If the delay in emptying becomes bad enough, the sinusoidal veins may not be adequately emptied by the time the calf muscles next relax. In that case there will not be room for much blood from superficial veins, and the pressure in these, which has been steadily rising, does not fall, as it normally does at this point.

C. Valvular incompetence

Though some believe that avalvulosis can be primary, breakdown in valves is usually secondary to involvement in the varicose process, or to having to withstand pressure that is abnormally high, or abnormally long sustained, or both. Inherited predisposition is also a factor. Fairly extensive muscular contraction, coupled with deep inspiration may momentarily arrest nearly all escape of blood from superficial veins into deep ones; though most of the time pressure in the great saphenous vein is high enough to overcome pressure in the common femoral vein. If there is incompetence of the valve at the end of the saphenous vein, however, whenever a wave of high pressure surges up the deep veins, retrograde flow into the saphenous vein will occur. In fact it has been observed to reach the ankle at phlebography.

Similarly, nearly all the larger perforating veins are guarded by valves. If they have given way, retrograde flow will occur whenever the pressure in deep veins rises above that in superficial ones in the area. When the perforating veins are of normal size very little flow will result through *them*. But these veins are particularly apt to become grossly dilated. Smaller perforating veins do not have valves, but for the pressure differences reached, only trivial blood flow will occur. No significant effect will result in the short time involved in calf contraction, provided these veins are of normal size. If they become dilated, however, they behave just like larger perforators with incompetent valves.

A normal venous system has a great many alternative routes by which it can empty. Likewise there are many different ways by which the superficial veins can empty into the deep. Thus the incompetence of just one valve is unlikely to have more than quite local effects. However, there is an important reason why the onset of incompetence in a valve in a perforating vein is so often followed by worsening of the clinical position. The reason is that breakdown of a 'perforator' valve has so often been preceded by failure of valves in a saphenous vein, usually the great saphenous.

Relative sizes of superficial and deep veins

This factor may call for some preliminary revision of related physics; for this does not seem to be widely known, or its relevance appreciated. The phenomenon is described in Chapter 1, no. 8: Tension and Laplace's law. It follows that if two tubes of similar wall strength come into continuity, the smaller tends to empty into the larger. (When the walls of the tubes have different elasticities or contractilities, this must also affect

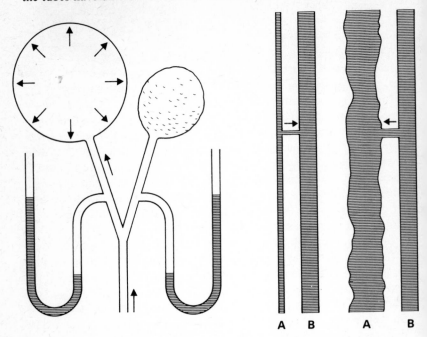

Fig. 22. *The Laplacian advantage described in Chapter 1, no. 8, affects the emptying of dilated varicose veins into the deep system.*
A: superficial. B: deep.

what happens.) Thus varicosity of superficial veins can greatly alter the efficiency of the calf pump by loss of what we have called the 'Laplacian advantage' and by loss of elasticity and contractility.

By Laplace's law, for a given pressure the strength of a vein wall requires to be proportional to its radius. This is another important reason why dilatation without proportional muscular hypertrophy can be so damaging.

Loss of the normal hierarchy of superficial veins will also do away with the normal Laplacian effect on blood flow in the superficial system.

Occupational factors

These do not operate during walking. Indeed, it is the absence of walking, with activation of the calf pump, that constitutes one of the most important occupational factors. Another is prolonged standing with unrelieved elevation of hydrostatic pressure in veins in the lower limb. Yet another is much repeated straining or heavy lifting, which raises intra-abdominal pressure and throws a heavy burden on the valves which prevent retrograde flow of blood from abdominal veins into veins of the leg. Worst of all is if one or both of the latter factors are combined with earlier ones, as they so often are.

Why varicosity is almost confined to the legs

We hold the reason why varicosity is virtually confined to the legs **not** to be, as usually assumed, that leg veins are subject to the highest level of hydrostatic pressure. Indeed, if it had been so, there is no obvious reason why the incidence of varicosity should be so different in the thigh and pampiniform plexus from what it is in the lower abdomen, and in the hand, which often hangs below the groin. Moreover, the incidence should have been significantly higher lower in the leg. Rather do we believe this to be the explanation. It would seem to us reasonable to judge that when man's ancestors first adopted the upright position, ample exercise of the calf muscles was the rule. But this keeps down pressure in the veins of the lower leg. And this reduced pressure is the one to which evolution would have adapted the leg veins. From an evolutionary viewpoint, very little time has elapsed since man first became an erect animal, and his leg veins can barely have begun to undergo the modification called for by the conditions of 'civilized' life. Under present conditions the veins of the leg alone have to withstand the substantial elevations of pressure that result from prolonged muscular inactivity, as well as the bursts of pressure occasioned by straining.

Turbulence

It has been claimed that varicose veins are caused by turbulence (Fegan, 1974). This would imply that the turbulence had occurred in normal veins before the onset of varicosity. Critical velocity (necessary for turbulence) is well above that of blood flow in veins, but it is not impossible that such velocity could occur very locally in close relation to a valve. However, this could cause varicosity only immediately beyond a valve, and varicosity sometimes starts just before a valve (see Fig. 23).

SUMMARY OF THE PATHOGENESIS OF VARICOSE VEINS

To summarize our concept of the pathogenesis of ordinary varicose veins, we hold that these do not have a single cause, and we feel that

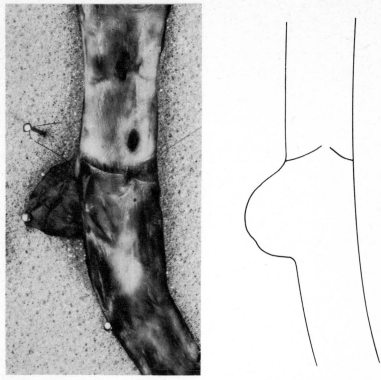

Fig. 23. Photograph of the inside of a section of vein, showing what appear to be normal, healthy cusped valves. An abnormal sacculation is seen just below the valve (upstream).

attempts to blame them all on one factor has bedevilled work in this field. We would accept, of course, that in different cases, different factors have predominated (not the same one in all cases, as some would have us believe). According to our view, the factors fall into two groups:

A. those that predispose to varicosity, and
B. those that precipitate, or hasten its onset.

These also determine that the disease shall be always progressive.

A. In this group we consider the usual one to be innate or inherited **local** weakness of vein wall, in proportion to the transmural pressure that it has to cope with here, in the circumstances of that particular patient's life, and having regard to any anatomical abnormalities present, innate or acquired.

B. In this group we include:

1. Old deep venous thrombosis, and the capillary and venous dilatations that have followed it;
2. Loss of valves whether congenital or acquired;
3. Loss of what we have called the 'Laplacian advantage';
4. Occupational factors.

Pregnancy and dietetic factors we judge to operate through the first group, either by direct action on the material of the vein wall, or through an effect on venous muscle tone.

In our view a very important manifestation indicating that the condition has already reached an advanced stage, is the presence of clinically obvious pathological circuits. These should not be regarded as a cause of varicosity, but rather as a step in its development.

CLINICAL FEATURES

For clinical purposes it is convenient to divide patients with varicose veins into those who came for treatment only for cosmetic reasons, and those who have more pressing symptoms.

Those who come because they are concerned about the appearance of their legs are almost exclusively women in their twenties or early thirties, who have noticed their abnormality only comparatively recently. Symptoms such as pain are usually absent at this stage, or nearly so, for slight symptoms may be admitted to on questioning. These tend to progress, however, and though at first they are confined to the region of the visible abnormality, they do not remain so. The earliest symptom is awareness of the presence of the vein. Later there is a feeling of local warmth and stretching of the skin. These symptoms may be noticed to be more evident in the evening, during hot weather, during menstruation, and in pregnancy.

On examination the varicosities are small or of moderate size, and the skin over them is normal, or near normal in thickness and mobility, though after prolonged standing it may be just lifted off the vein by a trace of oedema. Nevertheless, the skin over the affected veins may feel warm to the touch, and can be shown with a suitable instrument to be as much as 2° C. above what is usual. In most cases it is a tributary of the great saphenous vein on the medial aspect of the lower third of the thigh, or on the medial aspect of the upper third of the calf, that is first affected. The long saphenous vein, though not itself varicose, is often found to be distinctly distended in the thigh or in the region of the knee, sometimes with little saccular dilatations. There is rarely any clinically manifest involvement of the short saphenous system in this group.

In the second category are the patients with more pressing and better-defined symptoms. Whereas in the first group not more than segments of vein are involved, in this one, whole regions of veins (such as the whole area drained by one saphenous vein) are to greater or lesser extent diseased. In this group one patient in five is male. Typically these patients have much longer histories, often more of the order of 20 years. In nearly all cases both legs are affected, though seldom to equal extents.

In order of frequency the main symptoms are:

1. Swelling around the ankle after sitting or standing and disappearing over night in recumbency;
2. A feeling of heaviness in the calf;
3. Burning pain in the region of the varicose veins;
4. Itching.

Again all symptoms are worse in the evening, in hot weather, during menstruation, and in pregnancy. The symptoms are also exacerbated by certain kinds of straining or by prolonged standing. Night cramps are often said to be a symptom of varicose veins, but we have not found them to be commoner than in other patients of similar age.

On examination of a patient with more advanced disease, the first thing that strikes one may be that the superficial veins consist of a more numerous and denser network of large, intercommunicating veins than usual, and that the normal progression from smaller to larger vessels is lost. A tributary is often larger than the vein into which it opens.

The tributaries are without ostial valves, and the flap-valve mechanism described in the chapter on Structure does not appear to be operating. Abnormal directions of valves are often seen. For instance in the large vessel which normally connects the great saphenous vein to the lesser, the valves are often reversed, directing blood from the short to the long saphenous vein. Both large and smaller veins show evidence of disease. Also there are changes in surrounding tissues, particularly noticeable where the veins are normally near the surface.

Coppery pigmentation is common and is seen most in the ulcer-bearing area. It is derived from blood pigment and is the result of innumerable tiny haemorrhages from small blood vessels that have ruptured under the strain of prolonged over-distension. The staining may be punctate at first, but soon becomes confluent. Eczema is also common and may be dry and scaly or weeping and sticky. All these changes, both of the veins and of the surrounding tissues, are most concentrated on the medial aspect of the lower part of the lower leg. Oedema which at first is always pitting and reversible, is limited to the region of the ankle and foot. There is often fungus infection of the interdigital clefts and of the nail beds.

It has been pointed out that flat feet, hernia, and haemorrhoids are all common in association with varicose veins, but no more common, we hold, than in other people of this age.

In every case of varicose veins certain associated disorders must always be sought. These are: narrowing or total blockage of deep veins; incompetence of a valve with dilatation in a perforating or communicating vein; the state of the two saphenous veins, particularly of the valves at their terminations.

Sometimes patency or otherwise of the main deep veins is obvious from the clinical picture. The pathognomonic symptom of old femoro-popliteal thrombosis followed by complete obliteration of the lumen is bursting pain in the calf after standing or walking, associated with increase in volume of the leg. This symptom may persist even though venography has shown what looks like adequate recanalization. However, it is likely that there is still an important loss of distensibility of the vein, and that the valves in these veins, so important to proper function of the accessory pumps, are still incompetent. In the absence of this symptom of bursting pain and particularly if there are also none of the changes in the soft tissues described, then it may safely be judged that the deep venous system is working adequately. This may be even though there is a history of deep venous thrombosis, or strongly suggestive of one.

Retrograde flow in veins

Some writers have imagined (and even illustrated) normal, centripetal flow in deep veins continuing, yet retrograde flow occurring simultaneously in superficial veins. They have evidently thought the retrograde flow to be something that could occur all the time, where there was valvular incompetence. They cannot really have seen it happen for it is a physical impossibility. Just as forward flow implies a forward pressure gradient, retrograde flow implies a retrograde pressure gradient. For blood to flow from A to B in deep veins requires that the pressure at A shall be higher than the pressure at B. But for blood to return from B to A in some other vein requires that the pressure at B shall be greater than at A. Obviously these cannot both be so at the same time.

In fact cardiac action alone never causes true retrograde flow in the leg, and when retrograde flow does occur it has always been promoted by activity of one of the accessory pumps or by a Valsalva's manœuvre. For

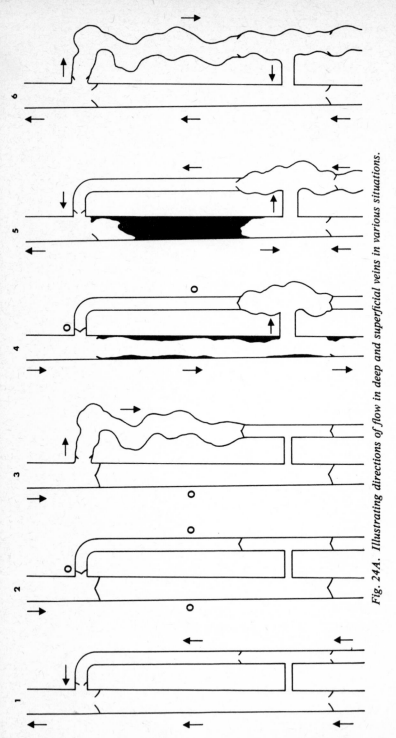

Fig. 24A. Illustrating directions of flow in deep and superficial veins in various situations.

1. Expiration. Normal.
2. Inspiration. Normal. (Pelvic valves not shown.)
3. Inspiration. Great saphenous incompetence and backflow.
4. Inspiration. Deep incompetence. Normal great saphenous. Ankle
5. Old deep venous thrombosis. Bypassed largely via superficial veins.
   Ankle 'blowout'.
6. As commonly drawn. Impossible simultaneous flow upwards in
   deep veins and downwards in superficial ones.

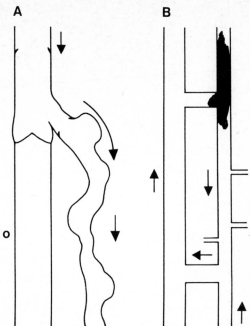

Fig. 24B. A *True retrograde flow. This only occurs during operation of an*
accessory pump; during inspiration for instance. The blood flows
retrogadely down a segment along which flow is ordinarily the other
way.
B *Apparent retrograde flow. Blood is flowing towards the heart, so far*
as the circulation is concerned.

example, if there are intact valves in the superficial femoral vein, but
incompetent ones in the great saphenous vein, and nothing to prevent
intra-abdominal pressure from being communicated to the common
femoral vein, a deep inspiration or a 'Valsalva' will cause transitory
retrograde flow down the great saphenous. It is more difficult for the calf
pump to promote retrograde flow except through a short incompetent
ankle perforator when there are also no functioning valves in the main
deep veins of the lower leg; but this only adds to the flow in the normal
direction in the great saphenous. The presence of a cough impulse in the
great saphenous vein, a very common physical sign in varicose veins,
would suggest that retrograde flow down the great saphenous vein when
straining, must occur. But it would be fruitless to look for retrograde flow
at other times.

Pseudo-retrograde flow

We have pointed out that **true** retrograde flow (that is flow away from
the heart, so far as the vascular system is concerned) is impossible,

except during activation of an accessory venous pump. However, **apparent** retrograde flow, that is flow downwards in leg veins, can occur continuously in segments of vein. Also, radio-opaque material can be seen, after injection at certain sites, always to follow the same downward route, before passing upwards. (It is following part of what we have called a 'pathological circuit'.) This is because, if a distal communication between a segment of superficial vein and the deep system becomes dilated and larger than more proximal communications, it may become the preferred route for blood reaching that segment from the tissues. Flow in the segment does, indeed, become reversed. Nevertheless, it is not truly retrograde, for it is still towards the heart so far as the vascular system is concerned. We consider it particularly important to recognize and eradicate these 'pathological circuits' as part of the treatment.

Clinical pressure changes

We have repeatedly confirmed that in recumbency as well as in standing subjects, there is a varying degree of elevation of blood pressure in varicose veins. In normal veins a rise in pressure is associated with increase of blood flow through the tissues and goes with the arteriolar and capillary dilatation that always occurs when there is increased metabolism and accumulation of metabolites. In varicose-vein subjects who so often have evidence of inadequate nourishment of skin and subcutaneous tissues, the elevated venous pressure is usually judged to be due to venous obstruction or inefficiency of venous drainage. However, this would be expected to be associated with increased de-oxygenation of the blood. But most workers have reported the exact reverse.

A combination which could fit such apparently incompatible findings is arteriolar dilatation, just as would be expected, but with closure of precapillary sphincters and true capillaries, the blood going instead through the arterio-venous capillaries. This would conform with our own views about venous pathology.

Pressure measurements (Fig. 25)

A single measurement of pressure in a superficial vein is of little use. But much can be learned from a tracing of venous pressure during activation of the calf pump. The apparatus required is expensive and the technique time consuming (about an hour for a doctor and a technician). It also involves a minor operation under local anaesthesia. It cannot, therefore, be undertaken routinely. It is of value particularly in specialized clinics in centres where research is going on, or where obscure cases are handled. Our technique is as follows.

First a dorsal vein of the great toe is cannulated, exactly as for phlebography (q.v.), using a gauge 16–18 polythene catheter. This catheter is connected to a Statham strain gauge via a system by which the tube is kept constantly perfused at a very slow rate. The liquid used for the perfusion is 2,500 units of heparin in 500 ml of normal saline.

The strain gauge is connected to a paper-roll recorder on which the paper is run at 100 mm/min. As the tube connecting the catheter to the strain gauge is filled with saline, the gauge must be kept level with the catheter. The recorder is 'zero-ed' in the ordinary way.

In a normal person the resting pressure in a vein on the dorsum of the great toe is a bit above the hydrostatic pressure, say 80 to 100 mm Hg (when standing). On rising on the toes no change is observed; but on relaxing the calf again, the pressure falls. A second lift reduces it some more and again with a third. About here the pressure levels out with a total reduction of 40 to 50 per cent below what it started at. If exercise now ceases, the pressure returns to what it was originally, in the course of a few seconds; that is more gradually than it was depressed by activation of the calf pump.

In venous disorders the reduction of pressure by activation of the calf pump is reduced in final extent, and is of more gradual onset. Also the return to previous resting level is more abrupt. The less marked change from normal is seen with ordinary regional varicose veins. It is more marked in cases meriting the name 'chronic venous insufficiency' and most so in postphlebitic cases. In fact, in some of the latter, particularly, if there are dilated incompetent ankle perforators as well, the pressure in the superficial veins may rise on contracting the calf and only fall again very gradually on calf relaxation; even then returning only to resting level.

In normals the effects are much the same whichever superficial vein is tested; but in venous disorders the abnormalities of response are far more striking in some veins than others, particularly in ones forming part of what we have called 'pathological circuits'.

All observations should be repeated, if possible under varying conditions, for often such things as the temperature of the room seem to make a difference to the response. (See Chapter 4: Accessory Pumps: The Calf Pump.)

Special clinical tests

1. *Test for adequacy of overall calibre of the venous system of the leg*

A tourniquet is applied as high as possible in the thigh of the patient while standing, tight enough to obstruct the veins, but not tight enough to

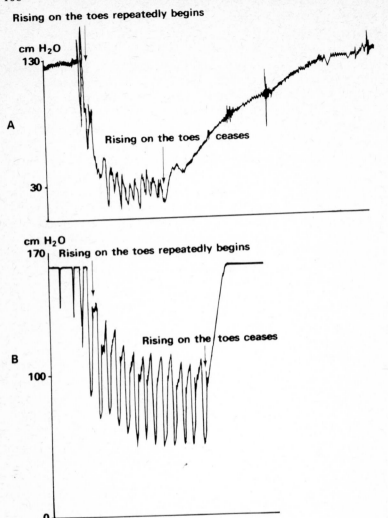

Fig. 25. *Typical charts of pressure measurements made as described in the text. A Normal. B Varicose veins. C Chronic venous insufficiency. D medial superficial system has been cannulated.*

interfere with the arterial pulse. The patient lies down, the leg is raised to about 45° and the tourniquet is released. The time required for the veins to empty is noted, preferably with a stop watch. This gives an indication of the adequacy of the calibre of the total drainage channels available to the venous system of the leg. It gives no positive information about the efficiency of venous drainage.

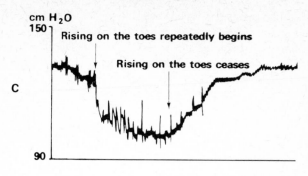

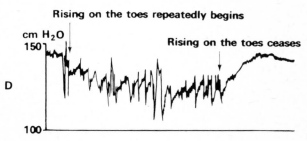

Tests for competence of valves

Tests which follow used to be carried out routinely. But the state of the veins should be the final arbiter in deciding what should be done. The competence or otherwise of individual valves may be of interest for records purposes. However, it has become doubtful whether the time the tests require could not, in a busy clinic, be better spent in some other way. The presence of a cough impulse establishes very simply the presence or absence of a competent valve between the palpating finger and the abdomen.

2. *Digital method (Trendelenburg's test)*

The patient lies down and the great saphenous vein is obliterated by digital pressure at its top end. An intelligent patient can do this better than can the clinician. While maintaining pressure, the patient then stands up. The vein takes a number of minutes to fill completely from the periphery and may be described as 'remaining empty' in a normal person without valvular defects of perforating veins peripheral to the groin.

If in spite of continued and correctly-placed digital pressure, the vein does fill fairly quickly (say visibly), it must have filled retrogradely through an incompetent channel connecting the superficial veins with the deep.

If the great saphenous vein does not fill, or if it does, before it is completely full, the finger over the fossa ovalis is removed. If the vein then fills promptly, the valve at its top end is evidently incompetent. This is the valve that most often gives way.

3. Triple-tourniquet method (Modified Perthes' test)

Three venous tourniquets are placed, one as high as possible in the thigh, and one just below the knee. If, when the patient stands up one or more of the isolated segments of vein fills rapidly, this segment has been demonstrated to contain an incompetent valve or valves. There is no point in carrying out this more tedious test, unless the simpler Trendelenburg test has been positive.

COMPLICATIONS

Acute

Haemorrhage

The most important acute complication of varicose veins is haemorrhage. Owing to their superficial position, their lack of contractility and the fact that the intima is adherent to the other layers and no longer free to coil up and plug a leak, quite minor trauma can cause dangerous bleeding. Though such bleeding is always easy to stop by simply raising the leg after lying the patient down, it can happen that nobody who knows this is present. In such a case, it is not uncommon for an over-large, inefficient dressing to be applied. Bleeding can then prove uncontrollable. Indeed, it can be, and occasionally is, fatal.

Thrombophlebitis and phlebothrombosis

Thrombosis in either superficial or deep veins is a common complication of varicose veins. A whole chapter has been devoted to the subject (Chapter 10).

Chronic

Skin changes

These are given under Postphlebitic Syndrome of which they are most characteristic (see Chapter 10).

Ulceration

See Chapter 11.

CHAPTER 9

Thrombosis and Thrombophlebitis

The fluidity of the blood is maintained by the delicate balancing of a number of extremely complicated enzymatically-controlled chain reactions. This balance is apt to be upset in favour of clotting by factors, some of which act locally and some generally. **Two different and microscopically differing reactions involving thrombosis occur in veins.**

1. The first is an ordinary, typical inflammatory reaction with the usual small-round-cell infiltration. As a primary condition of vein wall it is rare, for it is seen only as phlebitis migrans. But as involvement in inflammation of adjacent tissue, some thrombophlebitis of small veins must occur in every case of cellulitis (equivalent to the Continental 'phlegmone'), and even large veins used to be quite commonly involved (as in thrombophlebitis of the lateral sinus in mastoiditis). The clotting is secondary to the changes in the vein wall, and the clot is tightly bound to the wall from the start.

2. In the second and *common* variety the blood in a vein clots for one or more of a number of reasons other than local inflammation. Some act quite generally, though there must always be some local reason why the blood coagulates in one vein and not in another. A particularly important factor seems to be arrest or considerable slowing of the velocity of local blood flow. In this second category it is the clot itself that promotes reactions in adjacent tissues. There is none of the small-round-cell infiltration usually so characteristic of inflammation. (Though slowing of flow can promote thrombosis, total arrest only does so if there is at least microscopic injury to the vein wall.)

This second group includes the familiar deep vein thrombosis that plagues surgery and obstetrics. It used often to be called

111

'phlebothrombosis', which might have been a better name for all members of the group. However, another example is the commonly occurring spontaneous thrombosis of a varicose segment of superficial vein. Here the reaction in overlying skin and subcutaneous tissue shows all the usual clinical features of inflammation, and the name 'varicophlebitis' has become established. Another example is seen when a segment of vein has been isolated at operation, but inadvertently not removed. (Yet another is the thrombosed external pile.) In all these conditions, opening the vein and turning out the tense clot promptly relieves the symptoms, which are therefore presumed to be due to the pressure. One is reminded of the disproportionate pain and general disturbance associated with a tiny abscess in the tight pad of a finger, or with a subungual haematoma.

SPONTANEOUS THROMBOSIS IN A DEEP VEIN OF THE LEG

As a clinical entity bad enough to require treatment this condition occurs after 1 or 2 per cent of in-patient surgical operations, and in nearly half as many medical patients in hospital. It complicates about 0·05 per cent of pregnancies and follows about 0·5 per cent of childbirths. In 5 per cent of all cases there is no obviously related cause, though in over 90 per cent the patient was already confined to bed for some other reason when the incident occurred. Subclinical thrombosis, that is thrombosis that has been detected only by radioactive fibrinogen testing, may be twenty times as common. Some are subclinical only at the time of occurrence, for clinical evidence appears later; or they may be still unsuspected when first identified.

Factors known to increase the chances of deep venous thrombosis are: recumbency; more advanced age; and, less strikingly, female sex; certain circulating toxins and deficiencies, and blood diseases. There is a recognized association between clotting and remote malignant disease, as well as with operation, parturition, and pregnancy. Though a history of local strain not uncommonly accompanies an axillary thrombosis, it is not usually accepted in Britain that strain ever promotes deep thrombosis in the leg. The position about oestrogenic drugs and 'the pill' is not clear. If there is an association it is certainly a very rare one, and it seems to be confined to possessors of blood-group A.

A clot developing in the ordinary way in a vein, with some continuing flow, shows distinct stratification. There is a short, pale head containing many leucocytes, a very short, laminated neck, predominantly of thrombocytes, and a long, red tail, chiefly of erythrocytes. Such stratification is not seen in a clot that has appeared in an isolated section of vein in which blood has been stationary.

Spontaneous deep leg-vein thrombosis is a known risk of wakeful recumbency (with the knees straight). But it is also apt to develop after a long period with the knee tightly flexed as, for example, used to occur in a crowded air-raid shelter. There was also a condition known as 'steamer leg', which followed over-long spent in a deck chair, with the knee flexed over the rail. These were both often ascribed to kinking of the popliteal vein, assumed to have caused obstruction. However, no evidence of any such obstruction can be seen on flexing the knee during phlebography. The association of deep thrombosis and remote malignant disease and certain hormonal states are special cases which we shall not include when considering general causes.

The thing which bed rest in illness and states of knee-flexion described have in common is prolonged muscular inactivity of the legs. Spontaneous thrombosis does not seem to be particularly prone to occur during natural sleep. But this could be because people do not lie motionless during natural sleep. On the contrary, they change their position quite often. Patients lying ill in bed and awake, however, often tend to lie unnaturally still, almost as though they felt this to be expected of them as a condition of recovery. They also do this after childbirth, particularly a difficult one or one involving sutures.

However inactive the legs, some circulation of blood through them **as a whole** is maintained. But venous blood has a great many alternative routes, and the blood in one segment of vein can easily become completely stagnant. This must be particularly inclined to happen in intramuscular veins, such as the calf sinusoids, during muscular inactivity. And these are indeed the very veins in which deep-vein thrombosis nearly always starts. Accordingly, it is our view that the most important factor in the pathogenesis of deep thrombosis is muscular inactivity. To what extent advancing years operates through greater tendency to immobility, no one is yet in a position to say.

Thrombi in deep veins of the leg vary greatly in size, in site, and extent to which they resolve, persist, or increase. They also vary in symptomatology, though this depends a certain amount on the demands on the circulation in proportion to the extent of the block. In a recumbent patient, blockage of some 80 or 90 per cent of the larger veins may give rise to no complaint from the patient. This used to be called a 'silent thrombosis'. But like most vivid, metaphorical names, this is giving way to the weak but felt to be more scientific 'subclinical thrombosis'.

The thrombocytes play an important part in initiating the thrombosis, and the endothelium of the vein is particularly active in lysis. A great many factors combine to determine resolution, maintenance or extension. For though a thrombus often spreads either at once or later, it also has a strong propensity to undergo spontaneous dissolution. A fresh thrombus may be defined as one that is still reversible. In different circumstances it may be anything from several hours to a few days old. Since the introduction of heparin and other anticoagulants and fibrinolytic drugs, the designation 'fresh' has become applicable to many more thrombi, while others have been prevented from even starting, or getting beyond the subclinical stage.

CLINICAL FEATURES

Deep leg thrombosis is practically unknown in children, rare below thirty years of age, and uncommon between thirty and forty-five. After that it becomes increasingly common. Nearly all the earlier ones occur in relation to pregnancy or childbirth. When it occurs in a person already ill in bed, the severity of the thrombosis bears no relation to the severity of the pre-existing illness. Personal or hereditary predisposition may be apparent from a history of previous thrombotic incidents or family history. Deep venous thrombosis is also commoner in the presence of local or general conditions causing local slowing of blood flow, such as heart disease, ischaemic arterial disease, immobilization after trauma, and in varicose veins.

A thrombus in a deep vein often appears to promote less local reaction than it does in a superficial one, though there may be some mild general signs and symptoms, such as slight pyrexia, increased pulse rate and anxiety, leucocytosis and a raised E.S.R.

Symptoms may be singularly lacking, in spite of the old name 'phlegmasia alba dolens'. More often, especially with more extensive thrombosis, the pain is quite severe, as well as continuous. Or there may be intermittent cramps, or just a feeling of heaviness. The pain usually but not always, gets worse on standing or sitting up with the legs dependent; and it is relieved by lying down, or by compressive dressings or bandaging.

Swelling of the leg is the most characteristic feature, though only in the more extensive cases is there obvious pitting oedema in a recumbent patient. Increase in girth of the lower leg at calf level of more than 12 mm in a man or 15 mm in a woman, is usually considered significant. At first the swelling is confined to the superficial tissues. Later it may affect the subfascial planes, with resulting alteration of the shape of the leg. While the patient is flat the foot and ankle remain relatively free, but the oedema quickly shifts to dependent regions on standing. Except in the severer forms, the swelling disappears in a few hours in recumbency. The pain always starts before the swelling, either in the lower leg or in the thigh according to where the condition began.

Physical signs listed in order of diagnostic importance when present are:

1. Distended superficial veins in the affected area (as compared with the opposite leg).
2. Tenderness related to deep veins in the sole of the foot, or over the posterior tibial vein or the peroneal vein in the lower leg (the anterior tibial vein is very rarely affected), the popliteal vein, or the femoral vein. There may also be tenderness of a whole affected region on lateral compression.
3. Swelling of relevant soft tissues. For instance, in iliac vein thrombosis the external genitalia may be swollen, and there may be palpable swelling of tissues related to the rectum.
4. Involved skin may be slightly glazed or even visibly oedematous, as in 'peau d'orange'.
5. Cutaneous colour change. Pallor is the most usual, but sometimes cyanosis is apparent. A blue leg may become a white leg on elevation, or vice versa, a valuable sign when present.
6. Enlarged inguinal lymph nodes.
7. Relative coolness of the skin (after at least twenty minutes of exposure).
8. Diminution of the force of peripheral arterial pulses. More general features often present are slight elevation of pulse rate and temperature, and anxiety.

Among others, the following patterns may be recognized:

I. *Acute thrombosis of the lower leg*

This is a mild form with little tendency to spread. However, repeated small pulmonary emboli are apt to occur. Symptoms are not prominent in the early stages, and the condition is commonly missed until later. It is particularly apt to occur in patients who have varicose veins, or after childbirth.

II. *Acute thrombosis of the thigh and lower leg*

This is the well-known 'Phlegmasia Alba Dolens', or 'White Leg', or 'Milk Leg'. The condition is not so rapidly spreading nor so completely obstructing as in those of the next group. But it is very troublesome, is by no means free from danger, and can cause serious delay in convalescence after operation, or after childbirth. In most cases it starts in the foot or calf, and spreads proximally to the popliteal and femoral veins. On rare occasions it extends in the opposite direction after starting in the thigh. This is the kind most common after operation. In spite of the name 'Milk Leg', it is not the one most common after childbirth.

III. *Acute, massive venous thrombosis of the whole leg, with ischaemia (Phlegmasia Cerulea Dolens)*

This is a very rapid and severe condition. The marked tendency to extension, as well as to embolism, is evident from the start. Superficial veins are usually involved as well as deep. In fact the venous obstruction is so extensive that the circulation is virtually halted in the limb, and arterial blood cannot get in. The condition threatens the life of the patient, as well as survival of the limb, and treatment is extremely urgent. Characteristically, this is seen in elderly, debilitated patients, particularly with widespread malignant disease.

INVESTIGATION

Of the many methods of investigation available, three are of value in establishing the diagnosis of fresh venous thrombosis: **phlebography**, a **Doppler ultra-sound method**, and the **radioactive fibrinogen test.** We have not found the assessment of coagulability or of individual coagulation factors, or thrombo-elastography, or the measurement of retractability of a clot formed in aspirated blood, of any practical value.

Phlebography (see Chapter 7)

This is the most accurate and reliable method of recognizing the presence and position of a block, provided the radiographs are interpreted by someone with special skill and experience in this field, as well as having the necessary equipment. It cannot, of course, offer any clue as to the age of the obstruction, nor demonstrate its extent when the block is complete. Nor does it give any information (unless repeated) about whether the thrombus is extending or resolving. However, it can demonstrate patency in the relatively small main veins of the lower leg, as well as the large ones in the thigh; and it can often show incompleteness of a block.

Doppler method

The pencil-like Doppler-shift instrument is commonly equipped with two ceramic crystals. One is electrically activated and emits ultrasonic vibrations at constant frequency. The other receives the sound waves reflected from receding red cells, the received frequency being lower than the emitted frequency in proportion to the velocities of the receding cells. This change in frequency is the Doppler shift. The erythrocytes are not, of course, all travelling at the same velocity. Instead there is a 'profile' of different speeds across the vessel lumen. However, by sophisticated modern techniques these may be analysed, the diameter of the vessel deduced, and a picture, both temporal and spacial, of red-cell velocities obtained.

In leg veins information can particularly be obtained by observing the effects of respiration, and comparing these with normals. At present the instrument can be used in detecting ileo-femoral block, and arterio-venous fistulae. The method is in its infancy and is due for important developments (see Roberts, 1972). It cannot *yet* be claimed to have great clinical value and is used only for screening the largest veins.

Radio-active fibrinogen test

In this test use is made of the fact that as a thrombus forms it takes up fibrinogen from the circulating blood. If some of this is radio-active material that has been injected into the blood stream, the radio-activity of the blood as a whole may be seen to diminish. It can be sampled with a scintillation counter, over the heart for instance. At the same time radio-activity may be spotted where a thrombus is forming. The special advantage of this test is that it may be used to follow the progress of a particular thrombus. If a thrombus resolves, local radio-activity will diminish. At the same time the scintillation rate over the heart will be restored again. The given fibrinogen is labelled with ^{125}I, which has a half-life of about 6 weeks. Fibrinogen normally survives in the blood for an average of about 3 weeks.

The practical disadvantage of this method for routine use is that it is too sensitive, for it picks up even small thrombi, 90 per cent of which resolve spontaneously and do not justify full prophylactic treatment. On the other hand it gives the opportunity for especially thorough watching of threatened areas, and earlier institution of anticoagulant therapy for a spreading lesion, before it becomes dangerous to life or limb.

SUPERFICIAL PHLEBOTHROMBOSIS AND THROMBOPHLEBITIS

Two conditions associated with thrombosis of superficial veins are encountered in the leg, one common and one rare. The common one is a phlebothrombosis of a varicose segment; the other is a true inflammation of vein wall with secondary obliterative thrombosis, Phlebitis Migrans.

Phlebothrombosis of a varicose vein (Varicophlebitis)

A patient with well-established varicose veins, develops localized pain in the leg, but does not feel ill in general. On examination a segment of varicosity, usually of the saccular type, has become a hard, tender bar. The skin over it is hot, red, and swollen. All signs and symptoms subside at once as soon as the tension is relieved. We do not propose excision as a routine method of treatment, but ordinary surgical treatment for the varicose veins is not contraindicated in the presence of this condition. Accordingly we have, in fact, had occasion to apply such treatment in seventeen cases. In all we found the venous involvement to be much more extensive than we had judged it to be on clinical grounds. Also, though the condition is said never to extend to deep veins, in three the clot had followed medial perforating veins into the posterior tibial veins. It is true, nevertheless, that it may be depended upon that no clinically-manifest deep thrombosis will develop.

Phlebitis Migrans

This is a rare condition. It is a true inflammation of vein wall with the usual changes of an inflammation at microscopy. The clot is secondary to the phlebitis and is firmly adherent to the endothelium. It does not respond to anticoagulant or fibrinolytic therapy and is finally obliterative. Except that it attacks veins hitherto normal, the clinical appearances are similar to those seen in varicophlebitis. It also differs in that instead of predominantly affecting middle-aged women, this condition is seen almost exclusively in men between the ages of twenty and forty. The condition is also much more prone to extend or recur.

In this condition also, radical excision of involved veins has seemed to us a rational approach and has been successful in those cases in which it has been applied. Thus, in this lesion as well, we have had the opportunity to observe that the extent of the venous involvement has been much greater than would have been guessed clinically. Stripping is not practicable, but both saphenous veins are totally removed, as well as all affected tributaries. This is done through several small transverse incisions, from which the veins are freed by tunnelling up and down with artery forceps.

Phlebitis Migrans is said to be a precursor of Buerger's disease of the arteries. In a follow-up of twenty-seven cases from 5 to 15 years, we have not yet seen the suggested association.

CHAPTER 10

Chronic Venous Insufficiency and the Postphlebitic Syndrome

'Chronic venous insufficiency' is an expression introduced comparatively recently. It designates no more than a fairly advanced degree of trophic disturbances in the leg, believed to be due to inadequacy of venous drainage. Perhaps it has caught on because, while euphonius, it is conveniently imprecise and handy for those who have to avoid committing themselves to something more definite. However, our own dislike of the name arises more from the conviction that, even so far as it goes, it makes an incorrect assumption. For it suggests that the causative defect is diminution of drainage capacity of the venous system (as opposed to efficiency of pumping). However, we have already given reasons for believing that there is no important loss of carrying capacity. Indeed, later on the venous capacity is more often excessive, but ill-distributed. We have suggested that it has become *too easy* for arterial blood to go via certain arteriovenous capillaries, and dilated venules and veins, instead of via certain true capillaries of the microcirculation.

At one time, a popular name was the 'postphlebitic syndrome' and most people imagined that all cases were postphlebitic. But gradually it began to be realized that, as often as not, no deep thrombosis had ever occurred. Moreover, less severe deep thrombosis might be followed by no more than recurrent swelling, while other patients developed ordinary varicose veins; though a very few of the worst cases later showed changes never seen without earlier deep thrombosis.

In recent years, there has grown up a tendency to reserve the expression 'postphlebitic syndrome' for patients with unequivocal evidence of old deep thrombosis, and to call the other cases of severe trophic change 'chronic venous insufficiency'. Having made our protest and registered our reservation, we feel bound to retain an expression so widely used. We shall, therefore, restrict 'the postphlebitic syndrome' to the few cases with features seen only after severe deep venous thrombosis, while emphasizing that many cases of chronic venous insufficiency are postphlebitic.

Chronic venous insufficiency can also follow sufficiently widespread breakdown of valves, particularly the ones protecting the superficial system of larger veins from the deep. This has commonly followed their involvement in the varicose process or it may follow repeated attacks of thrombosis both superficial and deep (many of the deep ones having not been recognized as such or left firm radiological evidence of their occurrence). Another reason why deep thrombosis, even when followed by what looks radiologically like adequate re-canalization, may yet promote chronic venous insufficiency is this. The involved veins have not recovered their distensibility and contractility. The effect of old thrombosis that can be observed clinically is this. When tracings of pressure in superficial veins during activation of the calf pump, are made (see Chapter 8: Pressure Measurements), the usual reduction in pressure by some 50 per cent on contracting and then relaxing the calf, is much reduced or absent.

The postphlebitic syndrome was commonly thought of as a complex of signs and symptoms apt to, or even certain to follow any attack of deep venous thrombosis, even a single small one. But we have seen evidence in numerous necropsies that it is rarely after a single attack, but rather after repeated attacks, that the syndrome typically develops (Fig. 26). Each one obliterates a bit more of the venous system, superficial as well as deep. Accordingly, the postphlebitic syndrome should be thought of as often a manifestation of a progressive, still-active disease, rather than as a late result of an incident that is past.

A thrombosis, once started, may follow any of several alternative courses. It may, and often does, resolve completely, remaining subclinical throughout and not leading to any adverse sequelae at all. It may be associated with signs and symptoms as described in the chapter on acute thrombosis; yet these subside in due course, either spontaneously or in response to treatment. Or it may be followed by no more than a tendency to mild swelling of the ankle after particularly severe strain. Or the evidence of earlier deep thrombosis may be discovered for the first time at phlebography, or be deduced from the results of later pressure measurements in superficial veins. Sometimes, however, even occasionally in spite of treatment, all the signs and symptoms of acute deep thrombosis persist, or get worse, culminating in the classical post-phlebitic syndrome.

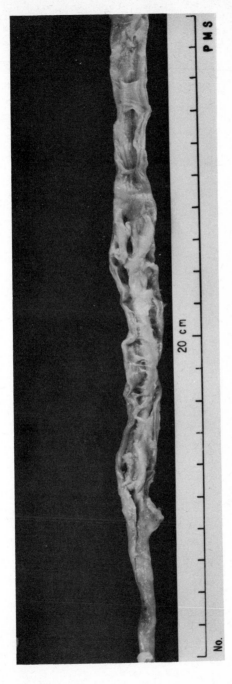

Fig. 26. Old thrombus, showing evidence of several stages.

In chronic venous insufficiency any combination of some or all the following signs and symptoms may occur.

1. Pain in the leg. This is commonly, but not invariably, present. It may have the character of a dull ache, or of bursting pain deep in the limb; or there may be only a feeling of heaviness. The pain is worse when standing or sitting up, and is easier while walking. In some more severe cases the patient also complains of pain in the ankle or knee joint. This is usually found to be associated with fibrosis of the joint capsule with limitation of movement, said to have been caused by venous 'stasis'. The condition has been called 'phlebo-arthrosis'. In a few patients a neuritic type of pain occurs around either malleolus, and is ascribed to neuritis of a nerve accompanying a saphenous vein.

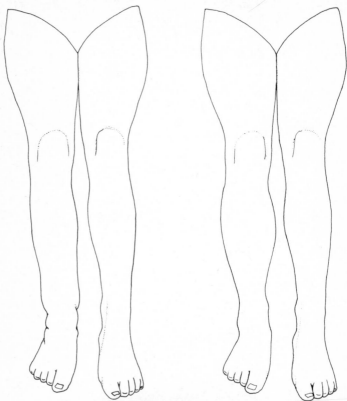

Fig. 27. *Shape of the leg typical of:*
 A. Chronic venous insufficiency, and
 B. The postphlebitic syndrome.

2. Oedema. This is the feature most generally present. At first it is reversible and markedly affected by gravity. In the early stages the oedema always pits on pressure, but later, when sclerosis and fibrosis supervene, it becomes firmer. Though it is mostly confined to superficial tissues, if much obstruction of deep veins has developed oedema may appear beneath the deep fascia as well.

3. Changes in superficial veins. Any of the changes described under 'Varicose Veins' may be seen. In addition in the skin about the ankle and the dorsum of the foot dilated very small veins may appear, of a dark blue colour (rather like spider veins), which disappear on elevation of the leg. Some of these may be more purple, as though their blood was partly arterial, or there may be brown spots which also disappear when the leg is raised. On the Continent all these features together are known as 'Corona Phlebectatica'. There may also be little punctate haemorrhages. These are seen at first as brown dots which do not change on elevation of the leg. Later they coalesce into larger brown areas of haemosiderosis.

4. Skin changes. Fibrosis and sclerosis occur. In some countries these are distinguished from one another. 'Sclerosis' is reserved for increase of non-cellular elements, while 'fibrosis' is used for multiplication of fibroblast cells and their fibrils. 'Atrophie blanche' is an expression used in other countries as well as France, for the small circumscribed scars left by ischaemic necrosis of the skin. They are often intermingled with a variety of papillomatosis consisting of little mounds caused by overgrowth and hypertrophy of the capillaries of the stratum pappilarium of the skin. The word 'dermatitis' is used to cover a great variety of skin changes from a thin, dry, glazed condition, to an exudative one with bacterial infection, or to a scaly eczema.

5. Ulceration. Every kind of ulcer described in the relevant chapter is encountered.

6. Induration of subcutaneous tissue. This presents as localized areas of fibrosis with harder foci of fat necrosis and the nodular remains of old venous thromboses. Both these may be found on the medial aspect of the lower third of the lower leg. They are rare elsewhere.

Recurrent attacks of thrombophlebitis are very characteristic and serve as a useful reminder of the continued activity of the disease. Fresh extension may be shown by no more than slight increase in pain and

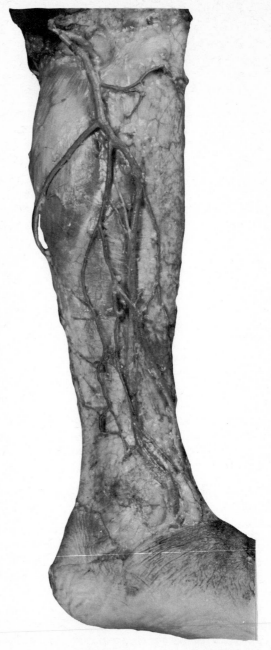

Fig. 28. *Showing plentiful large venous channels on medial aspect of leg, and relative sparsity on lateral aspect. Yet it is on the medial side that trophic changes chiefly occur, for it is here that the vital microcirculation is most easily by-passed.*

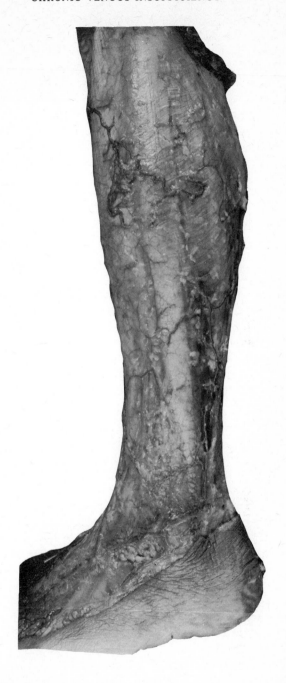

swelling, accompanied by general malaise, and sometimes by episodes of collapse, possibly due to small pulmonary emboli. The significance of the symptoms is often missed, both by the patient and by his physician, being judged to be simple exacerbation of his old symptoms, always made worse by excessive strain. These thromboses may occur in either deep or superficial veins. The condition is nearly always confined to a segment of a vein, is usually mild and incompletely obstructive.

We have not chosen to divide so-called 'chronic venous insufficiency' and 'the postphlebitic syndrome' into separate chapters, for we are satisfied that the sequelae of less extensive deep venous obstruction are no different from those due to any other form of venous disorder. However, very severe and extensive deep venous thrombosis can produce features that occur in no other condition. Typically these follow blockage of the iliac, the femoral, or the popliteal veins. In addition to any or all of the above manifestations in their severest forms, the following also occur in the postphlebitic syndrome.

1. Deep oedema. When there is oedema beneath the deep fascia as well as superficial to it, the deep is unlikely to be spotted. But now and again deep oedema is present alone. Then it gives rise to a characteristic picture, probably not possible to recognize from a description. The leg is generally distended, and there is a subtle change of shape, not a bit like the loss of shape of lymphoedema, but once *seen* never forgotten.

2. Widespread dilatation of the entire superficial venous system. This is present perhaps most conspicuously in the smaller tributaries, for these are not involved in ordinary varicosity. The main collecting trunks are thickened, fibrosed, and inelastic, but they do not display the lengthening or sacculation so characteristic of ordinary varicose veins. In fact these are far more reminiscent of the 'arterialized' veins of surgical arterio-venous anastomosis. Nor are the changes limited to segments of veins, as they are in varicosity. There is much evidence of valvular breakdown, and extensive retrograde flow.

These small veins are thin walled, distended, and closely adherent to the skin and adjacent tissues. Some writers have reserved the old name, 'secondary varicose veins', for these vessels. But we have preferred to abandon this name altogether, for it has been used with such varying meanings. We prefer to call them 'dilated veins of reticular type'.

CHAPTER 11

Venous Ulcer

By 'venous ulcer' we mean one which has followed a circumscribed area of gangrene of skin and subcutaneous tissue near the ankle, where a disorder of veins is believed to have been the fundamental cause. A venous ulcer never penetrates deep fascia to expose muscle or bone, though a little thickening of periosteum or even new bone formation may occur beneath it. Such an ulcer shows few signs of inflammatory reaction and if healing follows palliative treatment the ulcer has a strong tendency to recur. Though a venous ulcer is commonly related to a lesion of a particular main deep vein, it must surely be to a deficiency in an area of small superficial vessels that the ulcer must be more immediately ascribed.

Various local changes are commonly cited as predisposing factors in ulceration. These are trauma, infection and skin changes. But we would point out that these are all things to which the preceding condition of the tissues has rendered them particularly susceptible. It is indeed very common for the patient to attribute his lesion to some minor trauma, though the injury would rarely have had any noticeable effect on normal skin. However, all trauma increases local oxygen demands and must often be the 'last straw' in an area already on the verge of breakdown. Infection, bacterial, mycotic, or mixed, of venous ulcers is usual and helps to maintain them. But resistance to infection was already much lowered before the skin gave way. Skin changes are not so much predisposing factors to ulceration as earlier manifestations of the same deficiencies as later promote the ulcer.

THE CAUSE OF VENOUS ULCER

Observable facts are these:

1. Because of the free communications that exist between veins, venous blood has a number of alternative routes. For simple mechanical reasons, blood will always take the 'line of least resistance'.

2. If veins become obstructed, the ones which have to serve instead

become dilated and enlarged. Ultimately such enlargement can become quite gross, as in the abdominal wall in a survivor from inferior vena cava thrombosis.

3. A conspicuous feature of the legs of a patient who develops an ulcer after forty or so is the dense and extensively intercommunicating network of enlarged veins beneath the skin. As well as being so extensive, these veins are abnormal in that, unlike normal veins of this size, these ones lack ostial valves. Also, they meet the more proximal veins into which they drain, less obliquely than usual, so that the flap-valve mechanism normally formed by the obliquity of joining does not operate.

4. When previously small veins become sufficiently enlarged they begin to constitute the line of least resistance. When this becomes the preferred route for the blood, flow in the microcirculation of previously normal routes becomes progressively more reduced (as in the steal syndrome).

5. Most patients who develop ulcers have previously had a deep thrombosis (Dodd and Cockett, 1956), yet the ulcer often takes 10 or 20 years to appear after the main attack.

6. The early-developing ulcers, in the main, have the worse prognoses, and poorer responses to treatment.

7. Long-delayed ulcers nearly always develop on the basis of well-marked venous varicosities, fairly obviously related to the ulcer. Quickly-developing ones do not.

Current hypotheses for the cause of venous ulcer do not seem to accommodate all these facts, and particularly fail to explain No. 5, and why elimination of enlarged, bypass routes improves the condition of the leg and the ulcer. Accordingly we propose a different hypothesis which does both.

We accept, of course, that the fundamental cause of all venous ulcers is an inadequacy of venous drainage of the area which becomes gangrenous. The ulcer is an ischaemic one, owing to the diminished perfusion described. According to our concept, only the early-developing ulcers are precipitated directly by the obstruction. The later ones are caused more immediately by the largeness of the abnormal by-pass channels, which cause the blood to prefer these, and the blood-flow in previously normal channels to become inadequate.

CLINICAL VARIETIES AND CLASSIFICATION

As might have been anticipated from this description of the causes of venous ulcer, certain differences are to be observed between two main groups of ulcer. One group, **category 'A'** ulcers, are characteristically a disease of young people. Typically these ulcers start between thirty and

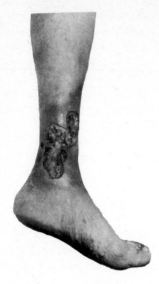

Fig. 29. *An ulcer of category A.*

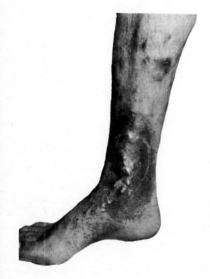

Fig. 30. *An ulcer of category B.*

thirty-five. Certainly most, and perhaps all of this group are post-phlebitic, and come on in a matter of months or a few years after the thrombosis, though only about 70 per cent still show unequivocal radiological evidence of one. Three out of four of the patients are women, and about half are obese, as well as having particularly thick legs. There are usually clinically detectable venous changes and occasionally well-marked varicosities, but seldom do these have any particular connection with the ulcer. The surrounding skin is extensively involved, showing induration and pigmentation at least. Oedema is usually substantial.

Venous ulcers in young people are commonest on the medial side above the ankle, but they differ from those in older people in being much less uncommon on the lateral side, or below either malleolus. These ulcers in younger people also vary more in shape and size and are occasionally painful.

In general category 'A' ulcers have a worse prognosis than those in older patients, and show a poorer response to treatment. Particularly is this so when the skin is dry, glazed, and tight; what Leriche called 'le

Category	Age Typical range	Deep incidence and thrombosis: How long ago	Varicose veins related to the ulcer	Proportion of males to females	Trophic changes in the skin	Oedema	Proportion obese	Proportion with fat legs
A	Young 30–35	? 100%	No Months or a few years	1:3	Bad	Severe	50%	Most
B	Older Over 40	1/3 Several or many years	Yes	1:4	Mild	Mild	Few	50%

peau trop court'. Ulcers in indurated, chronically swollen legs, but not with particularly tight skin, tend to become very large, and may even surround the leg. But these do not do so badly as might have been expected; for once healed, they often remain so for a long period. Two varieties do better than the general run. The first are ulcers that appear often quite soon after a lower-leg thrombosis. These ulcers tend to be small and dry. They are sometimes painful but have a relatively good prognosis. The other follows varicose veins of the reticular type (post-phlebitic). The leg is usually fat and also oedematous. This ulcer is often on the anterior aspect of the ankle, and has commonly been precipitated by trauma. It is not particularly painful, and responds well to treatment.

In the older group (say over forty), those of **category 'B'**, the preponderance of women is even more marked (four out of five). About half of them have fat legs, but only about one in five is frankly obese. Less than one in three has a definite history or radiological evidence of old deep venous thrombosis. All have varicose veins, and in all some of the varicosities are clearly related to the ulcer. Sometimes the ulcer lies over a dense haemangioma-like network of veins which have replaced other subcutaneous tissues; sometimes the ulcer follows rupture of a particularly thin, dilated vein. Indeed, occasionally the remains of such a vein is seen in the base of the ulcer. Sometimes the ulcer is just beside a single, dilated vein, which may be, but is not necessarily, a perforating vein. When it is so the ulcer is sometimes called a **'blow-out ulcer'**. But most commonly several dilated, thickened and tortuous veins leave the area of the ulcer in different directions.

These ulcers are uncommon anywhere but in the so-called 'ulcer-bearing' area on the medial side of the lower leg above the medial malleolus. They are circular or oval in shape, usually no larger than a 5p or 10p piece, and rarely painful. Skin changes around the ulcer are neither common nor severe, and oedema, if present at all, is mild. On the whole, ulcers in this group respond better to treatment than those starting in young people.

COMPLICATIONS OF VENOUS ULCER

Acute complications are seldom seen with a venous ulcer. One might have expected haemorrhage from an exposed vein, but in point of fact such a vein is more usually thrombosed. Acute infections, such as erysipelas, even tetanus, do occur, but are very rare owing to the adequate biological barrier set up in tissues adjacent to the ulcer. Malignant change (Marjolin's ulcer) is also very rare, but so common are these venous ulcers that most surgeons are likely to see a case or two of Marjolin's ulcer in the course of their professional careers.

DIFFERENTIAL DIAGNOSIS OF VENOUS ULCER

Their situation in the gaiter area, and their association with swelling of the leg, or with trophic changes in the skin, make the diagnosis of most venous ulcers straightforward.

The next most common ulcer in this region, which could be mistaken for a venous one, is an ischaemic ulcer, particularly when it appears in a leg already with varicose veins. However, these ulcers are commonest on the dorsum of the foot. They also occur on the lateral and anterior aspect of the lower leg. Ischaemic ulcers are associated with severe pain which, unlike that of venous ulcers, is made worse by elevation or by compression bandaging. There are also likely to be other signs of ischaemia, such as absence of posterior tibial or dorsalis pedis pulses, atrophy of the soft tissue of the toes, defective growth of the toe nails, absence of hair on the toes, and so on. Ischaemic ulcers are seen mostly in males over fifty years of age, with already-long histories of arterial disease.

There is also an ulcer of mixed origin, when both arterial supply and venous drainage are impaired. It often develops in the scar of a long-healed venous ulcer, being then most commonly on the medial side. The ischaemic symptoms tend to be milder than usual, and the feature which distinguishes this ulcer is its stubborn resistance to all kinds of treatment. Though feeble, pulses may all be just detectable. To confirm the arterial contribution, special investigation, such as oscillometry or arteriography may be necessary.

Ulcers of mixed origin, like pure ischaemic ulcers, also usually occur in males over fifty years of age. When seen in women they are nearly always associated with diabetes. Indeed, a glucose tolerance test is always performed when an ischaemic element is suspected. Diabetics are also liable to necrobiosis lipiodica diabeticorum. This manifests itself as several small ulcers on the anterior aspect of the middle third of the lower leg, with induration, and a tendency to run together. There are no associated venous or clinically detectable arterial lesions. Typically these are seen in fat women with relatively thin legs.

Another lesion presents as multiple small ulcers, mainly on the back of a thick lower leg in a young woman, with blotchy bluish discolouration of the skin of the legs. The ulcers appear after exposure to cold, and heal in warm weather. This lesion is called 'pernio' or 'chilblains' or 'erythro-cyanosis frigida'. It has occasionally been confused with erythema nodosum, though this is a lesion with induration, but little tendency to ulcerate. A rarity is a 'hypertensive ulcer' of which the aetiological connection with high arterial blood pressure is not understood. This is a 'healthy'-looking, shallow defect, with no exudate, but it is very slow to heal. They may occur over any bony prominence in the lower leg but mostly over the lateral malleolus of a younger woman with a long history of hypertension.

Ulcers which used to be common but are no longer seen in Britain are syphilitic or gummatous ulcers. They were apt to occur near the lateral malleolus, to be serpigeneous in shape, to be punched out with edges vertical to the surface, and to have what was known as a 'wash-leather' base. Gummatous ulcers were a lesion of the tertiary stage of syphilis. There are obvious circumstances in which they might become common again. The Wassermann reaction is positive.

Neoplastic ulcers which can appear on the skin are epitheliomas, with heaped-up everted edges, melanomas which may be, but are not always black, rodent ulcers with beaded edges, and metastases. Leg ulcers also occur in certain blood diseases such as polycythemia rubra vera, haemolytic anaemia, sickle-cell anaemia, and in ulcerative colitis.

CHAPTER 12

Lymphoedema, Non-vascular Oedema, and Lipoedema

LYMPHOEDEMA: DEFINITION AND GENERAL FEATURES

In his textbook, well known in its day, Aird (1957) used the expression 'lymphoedema' simply as a synonym for chronic oedema, and specifically stated that it was not necessarily of lymphatic origin. He listed thirteen varieties with thought-to-be-known causes, including four congenital kinds, and one 'post-phlebitic', in addition to an idiopathic disease 'lymphoedema praecox'. He also remarked that the harder one looked for a cause the fewer patients were left for the idiopathic category.

However, to many people lymphoedema meant, and still means, any kind of swelling thought to have followed failure of drainage of lymph. This would include a solid swelling judged to have resulted from clotting of an accumulation of liquid, as well as one obviously still fluid; for surely the only possible justification for use of the term 'oedema' for a solid swelling, is the presumption that it has previously been fluid.

Some have asserted that no oedema of lymphatic origin ever remains 'pitting' for long, but we have followed several cases of lymphoedema in which pitting can still be elicited after many years.

CLASSIFICATION OF LYMPHOEDEMA

Lymphoedema is described as **'primary'** or **'secondary'**, according to whether or not there is a known cause outside the lymphatic system. Perhaps prompted by the name 'lymphoedema praecox', some have subdivided the primary variety into an early and a later group, calling any that started after thirty-five years 'lymphoedema tarda'. But the disease does not fall naturally into such groups, and the choice of

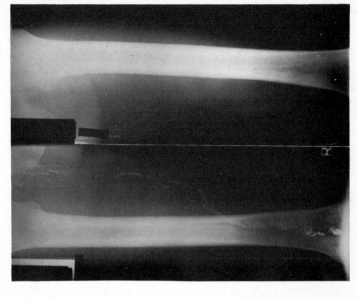

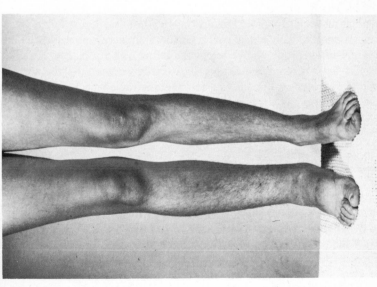

Fig. 31. Lymphoedema with lymphogram. The deep lymphatics are seen centrally, and the superficial at either side.

thirty-five was altogether arbitrary. Nor are different treatments used in early and late cases.

Secondary lymphoedema used to be divided into ones believed to have inflammatory causes, and so-called 'non-inflammatory'. The latter included such obvious promoters of lymphatic obstruction as surgical extirpation of lymph nodes, malignant infiltration of lymphatics, and high dosage irradiation. But the example thought to be most certainly inflammatory, is now judged not to be so after all. This was recurrent erysipelas. The oedema was thought to develop gradually with repeated attacks; but the disease always occurs in precisely the same place. Moreover, lymphography has always shown that lymphatic abnormality was already present when the first attack of erysipelas led to investigation. Accordingly it would seem that lymphoedema predisposes the tissues to this particular infection. Oddly enough, it does not seem to increase the incidence of any other infection of the tissues.

Lymphoedema has also been classified according to its site—proximal or distal, supposed cause, radiological appearance and so on, according to the feature which the classifier felt to be most important, but for our part we have found it most convenient to divide our patients simply into those more severely affected and those with mild symptoms, for only this has had any important bearing on treatment.

Many have felt the classification of lymphoedema to have been revolutionzed since the introduction of radiological investigation of the lymphatics. Radiological abnormality was described as 'hyperplasia', 'hypoplasia' and 'aplasia' (Kinmonth, 1954). These terms might have been thought to imply innate characteristics, but there is no evidence that they are never acquired. We adopt the terms with reluctance, for they seem to have become established, and we add 'euplasia' for the normal condition. However, attempts to correlate the radiological findings with clinical features have had disappointing results; though such correlations have seemed to be emerging from short series. Indeed, we thought we had observed some in our own series, early on.

THE CAUSE OF LYMPHOEDEMA

All lymphoedema was once thought to be the result of lymph retention, for it was assumed that any lymph that failed to get away by the lymphatic vessels would be bound to accumulate in the tissues. And before the nature of lymph transport was suspected, the only defect of lymph carriage envisaged was obstruction. It is now clear, however, that the chief function of the lymphatics in the limbs is the clearance of **protein** molecules, and **particles** from the tissues, the water of lymph being only that required for solution of the proteins and emulsifying the particles.

It is generally asserted that no protein at all gets back into the blood through the capillary walls, owing to the adverse concentration difference. But such a notion is not in accord with modern concepts of diffusion. The permeability of a membrane is a matter of the size of any pores in it in relation to that of molecules trying to get through. If there are any pores which allow proteins to escape from the plasma they must also let a certain amount back in the other direction. There is no doubt that a few thousandths of the protein that reaches the capillaries leaks through their walls. In other words, there is a small amount of **net** outward transfer. There must surely also be some back and forth diffusion of protein molecules. The transfer must be subject to derangement by alteration of the concentration difference, just as is the balance of water.

The total flow of lymph is but a tiny fraction of blood flow in the same period. The amount of water and crystalloids that diffuses through the capillary walls probably exceeds the total amount passing down the capillary (in other words, many molecules pass in and out more than once during transit of the length of the capillary). This extravasated or net outwardly transferred fluid is added to liquid produced in the cells as a result of metabolism and also diffused into the interstitial compartment. Of the whole, a few thousandths are used to make lymph. *All* the rest is reabsorbed into blood capillaries locally. It used to be thought that the proportion reabsorbed of that extravasated determined the volume left to become lymph. Now it seems obvious that this notion was the wrong way round. The volume of the lymph may be partly determined by the amount of protein for disposal, the water being simply the amount required for solution of this protein. After this amount has been subtracted from that extravasated, *all* the rest is ordinarily reabsorbed. (It was argued in Chapter 6, in Part I, that the volume of lymph flow is more probably determined by the activity of the transport mechanism.) Accordingly, any extra water left owing to diminished escape via the lymphatics can go instead via the veins (provided it is not held osmotically) without making any appreciable difference to the rate of flow of venous blood. Indeed, exercising a single finger would probably make comparable difference.

Inadequate lymph drainage would thus lead to a progressive rise of protein concentration in interstitial fluid. This would imply diminishing extravasation of protein from the capillaries and reduction of the barrier to their reabsorption. In fact it should be impossible for the protein concentration of interstitial fluid ever to remain higher than that of the plasma. The water of lymphoedema is often said to be held in the tissue spaces by the osmotic action of the retained protein. A fuller description is as follows:

According to the generally accepted hypothesis attributed to Starling, water and crystalloids are extravasated from the arterial ends of the capillaries because the blood pressure there exceeds the net osmotic pressure exerted in the opposite direction. At the venous ends, net osmotic pressure exceeds what is now the blood pressure. Therefore water and crystalloids are reabsorbed. Accordingly, *if* the concentration of proteins in the interstitial fluid rises and reaches parity with that of plasma, reabsorption of fluids would cease. Lymphoedema would therefore be expected to be progressive until skin tension was able to resist the excess of interstitial-fluid pressure. This is indeed what is observed clinically.

In no kind of lymphoedema has any trace of fluid been found beneath the deep fascia. A possible explanation for this could be that a higher level of pressure is required to produce oedema beneath the deep fascia. If our concept of lymphoedema is correct, there would be a limit to the pressure able to be developed in this kind of oedema.

Stagnant fluid with a protein content of the order suggested would be expected to clot. Crockett (1956) has indeed reported that he found the protein content of lymphoedema to be the highest of any. Moreover, he presumably tested oedema fluid from patients with still-pitting oedema, since no fluid can be obtained from a non-pitting oedema.

The nature of lymphatic obstruction

The lymphatic system as a whole has a pumping action (see Chapter 6). Like the heart, it pumps fluid from a region of relatively low pressure to one of relatively high pressure. (In fact, some creatures have what are known as 'lymph hearts'.) For this to be possible, efficient non-return valves are essential, and, as in the heart, **incompetence** of a valve can be just as disastrous as stenosis. The valves in the lymphatics are very numerous, but very frail. They are soon rendered incompetent by dilatation. In fact the worst kinds of lymphoedema are often found to be associated with a normal deep system of lymphatics, but a superficial system that is dilated and tortuous. Complete non-visualization of deep channels is a common finding in all kinds of lymphoedema. Yet with apparent total absence of both superficial and deep channels, quite moderate oedema is also commonly seen.

Effects of lymphatic obstruction

Lymphoedema is a chronic disorder, and some of its features, as with any chronic disease (and perhaps acute ones as well), are not so much direct effects of the diease as of efforts by the body to combat or adjust for more direct effects. One of the features of lymphoedema which one of us has discovered, may be such a reaction, and we can do no more than speculate about its purpose, and have no idea at all how it is brought about. Our observation has been that in lymphoedema there is *greatly increased blood flow*—by some 30 per cent. It was increased venous flow that we observed, and when we reported it to colleagues some of them remarked 'surely this is simply water that could not go via obstructed lymphatics, going by veins instead'. But this could certainly not be the explanation; for normal lymph flow is equal to but a tiny proportion of normal resting blood flow. Even if an amount equal to the highest rate of flow of lymph were to be added to the flow of venous blood, it would not make a detectable difference.

There can be no doubt, therefore, that what we have observed is *increased circulation of the blood through a part in which lymph flow is obstructed.*

We have also made the following observation. Lymphoedema was caused to appear in one hind leg of a dog by injecting the lymphatics with Neoprene Latex. As usual, the oedema entirely subsided in about eight weeks. The inferior vena cava was then ligated. Promptly oedema reappeared in the leg in which lymphatic obstruction had been induced, and became worse than it had been previously. Moreover, this time it persisted, and did not subside as previously. No oedema appeared in the contralateral, control leg in which the lymphatics had remained intact, and only the venous blood had been compelled to take alternative, less adequate routes Our suggestion, therefore, is that the advantage to the patient of increased blood flow would be the removal of some of the retained protein.

THE CLINICAL FEATURES OF PRIMARY LYMPHOEDEMA

We do not propose to copy out here descriptions of what others have asserted to be rare causes of lymphatic oedema, but to describe only what has been encountered in a busy 'swollen-leg clinic' and in specialized phlebological and lymphological practice. Nor shall we include any disease such as filarial elephantiasis, common only in certain parts of the world, and not seen in Britain. Instead we shall describe only the familiar primary lymphoedema, uncommon though this is compared with venous oedema. The lymphographic appearances already described cannot be correlated with any particular form of clinical disease.

There are two congenital forms, one sporadic, and one strictly familial, known as Milroy's disease, after the man who first fully documented it.

Lymphoedema praecox first appears most commonly in adolescence, 70 per cent starting before thirty-five. It attacks women more commonly than men in the ratio of 7 : 3. The swelling is first seen in a dependent area, usually around the ankle or the dorsum of the foot. It is always unilateral at first, though the other side is involved later in two cases out of five. However, it never becomes symmetrical. From the foot or ankle the swelling spreads proximally to the knee or groin, where it fades out. The rate of its inexorable progress varies greatly from patient to patient. It may reach the groin in months, or it may take years to reach the knee. Occasionally it extends so slowly that it remains confined to the neighbourhood of the ankle for many years, or even a lifetime. At first the swelling may be intermittent and relieved by recumbency, but this feature is soon lost.

A   B

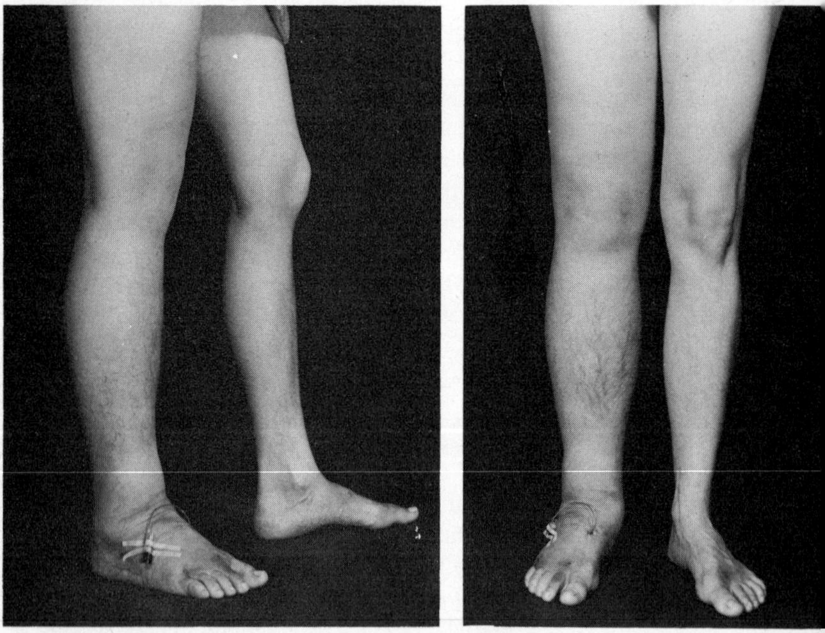

Fig. 32. A & B. Two views of the legs in a case of primary lymphoedema. The medial superficial system has been cannulated.

C

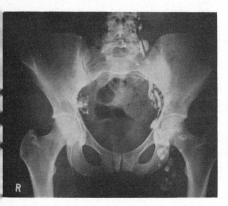

D

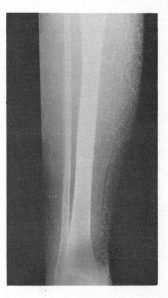

C. *Lymphogram of the pelvis, showing a normal pattern of nodes on the left. On the right no inguinal nodes are seen. Only a single superficial trunk is shown entering an abnormal lymphatic complex in the right side of the pelvis.*

D. *Right leg, showing hyperplasia of superficial vessels with dermal backflow.*

DIFFERENTIAL DIAGNOSIS IN LYMPHATIC OEDEMA

Even without radiological investigation, the exclusion of venous oedema rarely gives rise to any difficulty. A non-pitting oedema that does not respond to recumbency is immediately suspected of being a lymphoedema; and a non-vascular oedema is obviously out of the question. The absence of skin changes and of venous abnormality is also striking. Only a few cases of early postphlebitic swelling may require a little thought, though the history and the early response to recumbency soon settle the issue.

So-called 'lipoedema' is simply a symmetrical enlargement of the adipose tissue of the legs, extending to the groins. Often a woman accepts her fat thighs as normal, complaining only of the swelling extending from ankles to knees. The feet are not involved. Men with this condition often do not consider themselves abnormal at all, and this has led to a mistaken assertion that the condition is confined to women. There is often associated pain, and this tends to be worse in warm weather and at the menses.

One or two very rare conditions are apt to find their way to swollen-leg clinics. These include a diffuse form of vascular hamartoma. The overgrowth of vessels (very rarely the lymphatics) may be predominantly in muscles, joints, even bones, and commonly the skin as well. The whole limb is overgrown, the superficial veins are dilated, and there is pain. Also associated with overgrowth of the limb, but not painful, is naevus hypertrophicus varicosus or Klippel–Trenaunay Syndrome. In cirsoid or arterio-venous aneurysm heart failure usually dominates the picture. The neuro-fibromatosis of von Recklinghausen is hardly likely to cause more than momentary confusion.

Swelling due to hypersensitivity may also involve a limb, though only extremely rarely. There are always other allergic manifestations, such as asthma, hay fever, or allergic rashes. There is a periodic, familial form which can be dangerous.

COMPLICATIONS OF LYMPHOEDEMA

There is only one specific complication of either primary or secondary lymphoedema. This is recurrent erysipelas. This used to be thought to have caused the lymphoedema, but now it is generally accepted that it is the lymphoedema that has lowered the resistance of the tissues to this particular organism. For the disease always recurs in precisely the same area, and lymphography at the time of the first attack of erysipelas always shows that lymphatic abnormality is already present.

Clinical features of erysipelas

There is always a prodromal stage lasting 8 to 48 hours. There is tightness and itching of the area to be involved, and some general malaise. Later a sharply demarcated area of redness appears, with an advancing edge. Blisters may appear in the red area, and the itching becomes worse, associated with a feeling of heaviness. Some swelling of the affected area may be observed, and there is slight swelling of the whole lower leg. The red streaks of lymphangitis are commonly seen, but the regional lymph nodes, though tender, are not enlarged. At this stage there is usually high fever, headache, malaise, and vomiting. Abortive forms are also seen with less typical symptoms, but the diagnosis is not usually difficult, provided the condition is kept in mind. Untreated, the disease runs a varied course. It may resolve spontaneously, or there may be quite extensive areas of skin necrosis, or even a fatal issue, from septicaemia or heart failure.

Differential diagnosis of erysipelas

Erysipelas complicating lymphoedema is commonly mistaken for thrombophlebitis. On account of the severity of the fever, antibiotics have usually been given, but so often in small peroral doses insufficient for what can be a very serious condition. All the signs and symptoms respond within 48 hours to *adequate* dosage of penicillin.

NON-VASCULAR OEDEMA

By non-vascular oedema we mean an accumulation of fluid in the tissues in the absence of any apparent abnormality of either the lymph-vascular or the blood-vascular systems, excluding swellings with believed to be well-understood causes, such as the oedemas of heart failure, of nephrosis, of starvation, and so on. Indeed, no cause at all can be discovered on clinical examination or on routine investigation plus phlebography and lymphography.

In many of our patients the swelling of the legs has been only part of a general tendency to retain water, some other region being often more importantly affected. The condition is variously known as orthostatic oedema, premenstrual oedema, arthritic oedema, or geriatric oedema, according to any feature it happened to be associated with.

A certain number of people who have never before observed any tendency to swelling of the ankles notice it first after a long journey in a coach or aeroplane. In fact, in some larger countries where such journeys tend to occupy many hours, some people have had to give up plane and coach travel because of the discomfort and inconvenience caused. We have called this condition 'traveller's ankle', and cite it as another variety of non-vascular oedema.

The causes of non-vascular oedema

We believe this to be a group of disorders with a number of different causes. In one case several may have combined; in another, one has predominated or operated exclusively. One cause is constitutional, and seems to be a disturbance of the water-regulating mechanism, perhaps to do with the control of secretion of pituitary anti-diuretic hormone or of aldosterone. Another is associated with lethargy and may be related to myxoedema. A third only affects the feet and ankles, and appears to be due to inadequate exercise of the calf muscles.

Clinical features

Features characteristic of the first and last causes will be described, though instances will be encountered which do not fall obviously into one of these groups.

The symptoms of intermittent water retention are usually first noticed in the late teens, almost, but not quite, exclusively in women. Perhaps the condition is not really so rare in men, but they are less likely to go to their doctors with no more than a little transitory swelling of the ankles. The oedema is mild and pitting, gets worse as the day goes on, particularly with prolonged standing, but is made better by exercise, and disappears completely during the night. It is worse in hot weather and at the menses. It is bilateral and usually, but not invariably, symmetrical. As well as the attacks of oedema, there is intermittent oliguria, more than usual lability of body weight, instability of body temperature, and often intermittent headache. Mental instability is also sometimes observed, and a French team (Lagrue, Weil, Menard, and Milliez, 1971), who have called it a syndrome, claim that urinary infection is usually present. These authors have also reported a special tendency to extravasation of oily contrast medium in lymphograms. This is a thing we have not seen in any of our patients with non-vascular oedema, though it used to be common in anyone, with the old watery solutions. In about half of our patients there has been evidence of unusually rapid clearance of contrast medium in both phlebograms and lymphograms. This has suggested abnormally copious resting volume flow of both blood and lymph. Characteristically, this 'supernormal' flow was most evident in the worst cases.

Another variety of non-vascular oedema is instanced by traveller's ankle. This is seen more in older people and, though commoner in women, is also common in men.

Traveller's ankle

One of us recently wrote to medical journals (Johnson, 1973a, b and c) reporting a condition which, it seemed, had not been described before, and which has turned out to be much commoner than had been guessed. Traveller's ankle is a pitting oedema of the ankles, coming on towards the end of a long journey in a coach or aeroplane, and associated with a varying degree of discomfort or pain. Those travelling by train or car seem to be relatively immune. A characteristic feature of the condition is that it subsides altogether in a few hours of recumbency **or of walking**. Indeed, this distinguishes the condition from another which comes on less commonly in identical circumstances. This is spontaneous deep venous thrombosis.

Differentiation from deep venous thrombosis

Deep venous thrombosis, as well as being apt to develop in patients lying very still for long periods in hospital, is also occasionally seen after overlong spent with the knees flexed. It used to occur sometimes on board ship in a passenger who had been sitting with legs flexed over the rail of a deck chair (steamer leg), and it became familiar during the war after a night in an over-crowded air-raid shelter (shelter leg). The most important distinguishing point is that in deep venous thrombosis the pain, which is often quite severe, always precedes the swelling, while in traveller's ankle it is the other way about.

Steamer leg and shelter leg, as well as some cases of deep venous thrombosis occurring in hospital, were often ascribed to imagined obstruction of the popliteal vein by kinking behind a flexed knee, though if this had occurred it would not have explained why the clotting nearly always started in intramuscular veins. Moreover, when the knee is flexed during phlebography, no evidence of obstruction can be seen in the popliteal vein. Exactly the same applies to traveller's ankle. Our own view is that in both conditions the essential feature they all have in common is not flexion of the knee, which we believe to be unimportant, but inadequate exercise of the calf pump. This would explain why traveller's ankle seldom occurs in passengers in trains or cars, for these are able to move their legs now and again, while most coach and plane passengers are not. It is our belief that inadequate exercise of the calf pump is an important contributory factor in many forms of non-vascular oedema, and may be the main one in arthritic oedema and geriatric oedema.

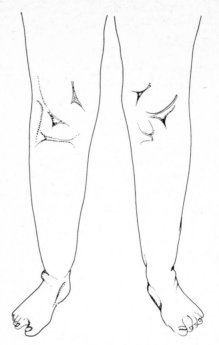

Fig. 33. Lipoedema or lipidosis.

LIPOEDEMA OR LIPIDOSIS

Lipoedema is a diffuse enlargement of the subcutaneous fatty tissue of the lower limbs. No abnormality is noticed until the patient's body undergoes the usual changes associated with puberty. At the upper end the swelling has no sharp limit, but at the ankle it ends abruptly. The hollows on either side of the Achilles tendon are filled with fat, and shapeless, but the malleoli and the whole of the rest of the foot are normal. The condition is absolutely symmetrical. Above the waist these patients seem disproportionately slim. The condition is often thought to be confined to women but it is by no means unknown in men. However, in them it does not cause the profound psychological trauma that it does in women. Later in life, as the tissues become flabby, the abnormal fat tends to accumulate in sagging masses. Perhaps it will be already obvious to the reader that 'lipoedema' is a misnomer as well as being far too much like the name 'lymphoedema'. We should prefer 'Lipidosis'.

For the purpose of management, the stage of regionalization may be given a separate status; for, while nothing can be done in the early stages, the later regionalized stage lends itself to excisions.

ADDENDUM TO PART II

Leg Swelling in Pregnancy

Swelling of the leg coming on during pregnancy or the puerperium will be considered under four headings:

1. Deep venous thrombosis;
2. Varicose veins and spider veins;
3. Lymphoedema;
4. Non-vascular oedema.

1. Deep venous thrombosis

According to Daniel (1969), spontaneous deep venous thrombosis bad enough to require full treatment occurs in about one in 2,500 pregnancies or in early post-partum periods. However, in spite of being rare, it is far the most important cause of leg swelling in this period, because it is the only one dangerous to life and because of the great urgency of diagnosis and treatment. In most cases the onset is sufficiently sudden and the pain, which always comes before the swelling, is sufficiently severe to alert the patient's medical attendants. However, in a few the condition comes on less dramatically. In pregnancy or a labour ward, almost any pain or leg swelling is apt to be ascribed by the patient and others to her physiological condition, and there is a real danger that in a deep venous thrombosis of insidious onset the only time for effective treatment will be allowed to slip by.

The first rule should be that any sudden leg pain or swelling in pregnancy or the puerperium must be assumed to indicate deep venous thrombosis until proved not to do so. The best management consists in very frequent clinical examination (say 3 or 4 hourly) until the diagnosis is certain. If deep thrombosis continues to be suspected, the diagnosis may be confirmed by phlebography, for this examination is not contra-indicated in pregnancy as the radio-isotope test is.

147

2. Ordinary varicose veins

There is a strong tendency for ordinary varicose veins to appear or become worse during pregnancy, and this is assumed to be because of some hormonal effect on the vein walls. It occurs too early in pregnancy to be attributable to mechanical obstruction of veins in the abdomen by the enlarging uterus, or by increased intra-abdominal pressure. Incidentally, the assumption that intra-abdominal pressure rises during pregnancy has been shown to be mistaken.

The varicose veins of pregnancy differ from other varicose veins in only one respect. This is that they largely subside after parturition, which has an obvious bearing on management. This tendency to disappear is most marked in the smaller tributaries and in spider veins, and less so in main veins and their immediate tributaries. The varicose veins of pregnancy may be accompanied by moderate or quite severe swelling, and they may become more painful than previously. Both these features also improve after parturition.

Spider veins or microvarices tend to appear in patches some 3 to 10 cm across, anywhere on the lower limb. They are of bluish colour. They usually itch. They are not the cause of any leg swelling that accompanies them, which must therefore be considered to be non-vascular oedema (if not, of course, due to deep venous thrombosis, or to ordinary varicose veins).

3. Lymphoedema

We have seen 5 patients in whom lymphoedema may have been precipitated by pregnancy, though 4 of them admitted to earlier occasional ankle swelling. In 2 of 19 patients with frank lymphoedema at the start of pregnancy, the swelling became worse; but in 3 it became slightly better. Most lymphoedematous women during pregnancy have an increased feeling of heaviness in the legs, and think the swelling has got larger, though this seldom amounts to a clinically detectable increase. Moreover, it affects both legs equally, even though one was previously normal. We have concluded that it is due to mild superadded non-vascular oedema.

4. Non-vascular oedema

Swelling of the legs without detectable abnormality of veins or lymphatics is the commonest kind in pregnancy. It is usually believed to be hormonally induced and to be part of a general tendency to retain water. Impairment of renal function is also common in pregnancy. The swelling is bilateral and symmetrical. It causes little in the way of symptoms. The swelling quickly responds to elevation. The tendency to leg swelling disappears after parturition.

PART III

Treatments
and their rationales, indications, contraindications and complications

CHAPTER 13

The Treatment of Oedema of the Leg

Treatments for oedema of the leg fall into two groups: those designed to combat oedema along general lines, by encouraging its absorption and discouraging further formation; and those aimed more specifically at the cause. Treatments directed at the oedema itself approach the problem through the four pressures concerned in fluid extravasation and reabsorption through the capillaries (see Chapter 5: Formation and Disposal). They will follow as many as possible of the following lines:

1. Increasing the effective pressure of fluid in the interstitial compartment. This is achieved by the application of external compression, usually with an elastic bandage or appliance.

2. Reducing intracapillary blood pressure. Far the most effective way to do this is by elevating the limb. In fact, if the leg is raised above the heart, pressure in the veins may fall below atmospheric pressure, and the veins will collapse. Pressure in the capillaries is reduced accordingly. Other methods which reduce peripheral venous pressure, and through it the capillary pressure, are exercise of the muscle and respiratory pumps by calf and thigh exercises, and by deep breathing.

3. Diminishing the osmotic pressure of the oedema fluid. This is believed to depend largely on the protein content. Proteins are ordinarily cleared from the interstitial compartment in lymph. Anything that increases lymph flow is therefore recommended in oedema. Other methods designed to operate through advantageous manipulation of chemical linkages or of the physical state of the material, probably await discovery. The flow of lymph is encouraged by exercise and by massage. Muscle exercise increases lymph formation and may not increase lymph transport more than enough to cope with these extra requirements. Massage, however, more probably works largely if not entirely through improvement of lymph transport. Many specialists in physical medicine now say that there is no evidence that massage affects oedema. This is

153

not our impression, but we have not had the opportunity to conduct the necessary controlled experiment.

4. Increasing the osmotic pressure of the plasma. Such extreme methods as the administration of intravenous plasma concentrate will obviously rarely be called for, though diuretics may occasionally be considered. In fact it has been demonstrated by one of us (Pflug, 1973) that some, if not all, of the many patent medicines advertised for the treatment of oedema of the leg promote diuresis, and do not have any selective action on oedema of the legs. This is not to say that they do not improve the condition for which they are advertised, for they do.

In summary, therefore, the treatment of oedema along general lines may include elevation, compression, exercise of the limb, massage, breathing exercises, and diuretic and other anti-oedematous drugs.

ELEVATION

Elevation is widely believed to improve venous drainage from the leg by allowing venous blood to flow downhill instead of up, but this is quite mistaken. As explained in Chapter 1, no. 11, the vascular system is a circuit or syphon. In such a system it makes no difference to the energy requirements whether the contents are flowing first up then down, or first down then up, or staying all the time on the same level. The extra pressure head needed to lift blood from the feet in the standing position is exactly matched by the extra pressure in all vessels in the feet for gravitational reasons when standing.

This is true whether the system is rigid or flexible. But the fact that the vascular system is elastic introduces another factor which actually operates the other way from that popularly believed. Because hydrostatic pressure in all vessels in the feet is increased on standing these vessels dilate somewhat. An effect of this is disproportionately to reduce their resistance to flow ((in proportion to calibre $\div$ 2)^4). *Thus it is when the legs are dependent and not when they are elevated that venous drainage is most easy.*

It is true that when a leg is elevated there is an immediate increase in volume flow in the veins, as one of us has confirmed with a flow meter, but this only represents blood being got rid of from the veins as they constrict. The increase very soon slows and the flow returns to equality with arterial entry, now reduced from what it was in the dependent position.

There is no corresponding effect on lymph flow, for there are no hydrostatic gravitational effects on lymph or on interstitial fluid. This is because the lymph vessels, even the smallest, are closely valved right down to the initial lymphatics at the start of the system, coupled with the great slowness of flow of lymph, and the fact that a row of valves are therefore never open simultaneously; also there is no continuous body of liquid in the interstitial compartment (see Chapters 5 and 6).

However, elevation is the best of all treatments for oedema, though not for the reason popularly supposed.

The reason why elevation is so effective in pitting oedema is because it is far the most efficient method of reducing intracapillary pressure, and this greatly outweighs its adverse effect on venous flow.

For the reasons described in Chapter 5 this discourages further formation of oedema and encourages absorption of the oedema already present, into the capillaries.

Oedema fluid, at least that of venous origin, does appear to shift around the body under the influence of gravity, to the most dependent areas. But it does not remain subcutaneous and therefore visible while it does so. There seems to be no doubt that it absorbs into the blood stream where capillary pressure is relatively low, and is redeposited where capillary pressure is highest. The reason why elevation is so much less effective in lymphoedema is discussed in Chapter 12.

Mechanically, elevation is much superior to compression, for a mere 15 cm (6 in.) of elevation is mechanically equivalent to extra tension on a 15 cm (6 in.) bandage of about 500 g (say 1 lb.), which is more than should be applied to the leg of a recumbent patient.

A practical point in the control of elevation is to bear in mind that it is elevation in relation to the whole of the rest of the patient's body that matters. So often a thoughtless nurse, or one who has not understood the purpose of elevation, undermines the effect by propping up the patient in bed. There is no harm in allowing a pillow for the head, particularly if the leg is further raised on pillows.

In a review of work on the control of circulation during exercise (Bevegard and Shepherd, 1967), it was pointed out that 'elevation of the arm would reduce perfusion pressure'. Perfusion pressure is the difference between arterial pressure and venous pressure of the part. Elevation does, indeed, diminish arterial pressure. However, up to the phlebostatic level it also diminishes venous pressure to an exactly equal extent. It therefore has no effect whatever on perfusion pressure. Above the level of venous collapse syphonage does not work (see Chapter 1, no. 11), for veins cannot conduct sub-ambient pressure. Instead, they collapse and close. Even without syphonage there is still plenty of arterial pressure to lift arterial blood to the elevated finger-tips, and maintain slow perfusion. But the perfusion pressure in the forearm muscles, for instance, is likely to be reduced by about 20 per cent, with a similar reduction in perfusion *rate*.

A

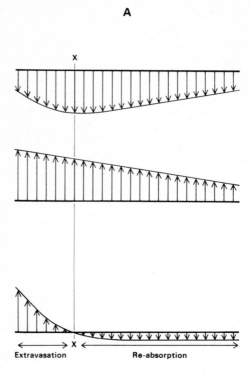

Fig. 34. *The effects of conservative treatment. As in Fig. 11, the graphs represent from top to bottom, changes in net osmotic pressure, transmural hydraulic pressure, and net diffusion. A. is normal, and shows balanced extravasation and reabsorption. B. shows the effects of elevation or compression, both of which decrease transmural hydraulic pressure, the first by reducing capillary pressure, the second by raising interstitial-fluid pressure. C. shows the effects of diuretics on intravenous plasma concentrates. Both increase the osmotic pressure of the plasma. All four cause absorption to exceed extravasation.*

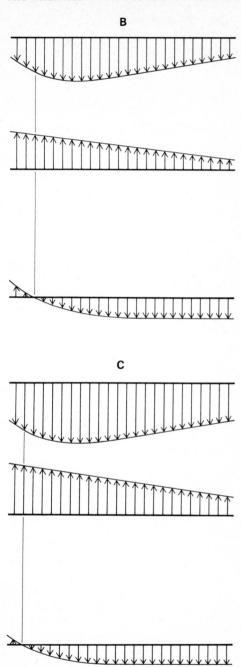

Much more important than this, however, is the effect of reduction of hydrostatic pressure on vascular calibre, for reduction of this by only 10 per cent must be expected to diminish perfusion some 30 or 40 per cent (34 per cent for a Newtonian fluid like plasma).

COMPRESSION

Compression was tried empirically and found to be effective in many cases of swelling of the leg, long before anything was understood about its mode of operation. In fact it works by increasing the effective interstitial-fluid pressure, so inclining the four pressures (see Chapter 5: Formation and Disposal) towards preponderance of reabsorption over extravasation of fluids into or out of the capillaries. It seems to be little appreciated how very different are the amounts of compression that can be safely and painlessly applied to the legs of standing and of recumbent patients.

In the management of varicose veins, when compression is used, the object may be to empty the superficial veins, and to do this may require a degree of compression at least equal to the hydrostatic pressure in them at the moment, and this may be much more than is either necessary or comfortable in recumbency.

It would seem unlikely that the clinician would ever wish to risk interfering with the microcirculation. We would therefore urge that any pressure over that likely to be encountered in the capillaries should be shunned. We would suggest a pressure of 10 mm Hg as the highest that should be allowed at heart level. On standing (not walking) the pressure in the capillaries of the foot rises some 80 or 90 mm Hg, and obviously much heavier compression will be both safe and painless.

To calculate the compression achieved by any particular bandage tension, Laplace's law for tubes would be used. $P = T/R$, where P is the pressure achieved, in cm H_2O, T is the bandage tension, in g weight/cm, and R is the radius of curvature of the surface being bandaged, in cm. Thus for an average ankle radius of 4 cm, a pressure of 10 mm Hg would correspond with a bandage tension of 54·4 g weight per cm. Allowing for the usual 50 per cent overlap of the bandage, this would amount to 408 g (14 oz.) on a 15 cm (6 in.) bandage. This is what is exerted by a new crêpe bandage at moderate extension. (At **full** stretch it can exert five times that; but the tension eases off very quickly after application.)

Such moderate tension is very difficult to apply with anything heavier or more elastic than a crêpe bandage. No wonder that patients who have had a heavier compressive bandage applied, without instructions to remove it at night, experience such severe pain, which they find they can relieve only by getting up and walking about. For a recumbent patient we therefore advise moderate extension of a crêpe bandage. For ambulant patients if firmer bandaging is employed we would urge that it be removed at night, and reapplied immediately before rising every morning. For the same reason we are strongly opposed to the adhesive elastic bandage which is specifically designed to be left on for long periods, and will obviously apply practically the same compression day and night.

It is usual to advise that the tension on an elastic bandage should become less as bandaging proceeds up the leg. The rationale for this in a recumbent patient is dubious, but in the leg of a standing patient the pressure in the veins of the foot is likely to be twice what it is at the groin. However, the advice must have taken no cognisance of the fact that the compression exerted by an elastic bandage, as well as varying directly with the tension, varies inversely as the radius of curvature of the bandaged surface. The radius of curvature in the thigh is usually more like three times what it is at the ankle. Thus if the bandage is applied with even tension from foot to groin, the difference in venous pressure at the two ends will have been more than compensated for.

A new method of compression has been introduced by one of us (J.P.) and is now available. It was used first in the hope that by improving the circulation through the calf sinusoids of recumbent patients the incidence of post-operative thrombosis might be reduced. It was unexpectedly successful, and is now being used with success for other purposes as well. The machine is like a plastic legging with an inflatable lining. It buttons right down the front, exposing the base of the toes. With its help intermittent air pressure is applied to the leg. Each pulse of pressure empties the superficial veins in the area embraced by the boot, and probably some of the deep veins as well. Because of the orientation of the valves this blood is prevented from flowing back into the lower leg during the period of relaxation of pressure, and a pumping action results (see Appendix, no. 9).

CHAPTER 14

The Treatment of Varicose Veins

Some of the symptoms associated with varicose veins arise, not from the varicosities themselves, but from an underlying lesion which has often preceded the varicosities. In fact it may have largely promoted them. Treatment of varicose veins can hardly be expected, for instance, to cure the bursting pain of deep venous obstruction. Symptoms attributable to the varicosities themselves are relieved by keeping the affected veins empty. This can be done by *compression*, by *sclerotherapy*, or by *surgery*.

THE CHOICE BETWEEN CONSERVATIVE AND SPECIFIC TREATMENT

Compression has no curative effect on varicose veins, relieving the symptoms only so long as it is applied. Compression can therefore represent only procrastination of definitive methods, or a deliberate choice of a form of management which, at the best, can only maintain the patient in his present state for the rest of his life. If the patient is less fortunate he may suffer one of the complications from which he has continued to be at risk. How many patients can have appreciated this when they were induced to adopt this line of management?

Compression is non-selective, for it cannot be applied to less than the whole of the superficial venous system of the area bandaged. It is also likely to affect some of the deep veins as well, and may interfere with the microcirculation. Compression is a constant nuisance, requires frequent attention, and can be very uncomfortable, especially in hot weather. However, it involves no irrevocable decisions and is less alarming to the timid patient. It is often felt by the patient to offer the advantages of simplicity and cheapness both in money and time. Compression controls oedema as well as pain, and if properly maintained may prevent complications. Even though veins in the thigh are involved, a compressive appliance worn only below the knee will usually relieve the symptoms, and may therefore be recommended in hot weather.

A great variety of compressive dressings are available, both wet and dry. The wet ones are particularly favoured by some when an ulcer is present. Then there is a great range of elastic bandages of varying strengths and direction of elasticity, any of which are probably suitable for day-time use. We are opposed only to the adhesive elastic bandage, specifically designed to remain on for periods of several weeks, and therefore applying similar pressure day and night, a principle we deplore. The most suitable appliance for varicose veins is, in our view, the elastic stocking. It requires no special skill or judgement in application. It does not slip and suddenly require re-application. It can be left off at night or for bathing. Moreover, if compression is to be used at all for varicose veins, such management is likely to be prolonged, and this is another reason for avoiding more troublesome or messier applications. Elastic stockings have only one drawback. They are ordered 'to measure', but are not usually specially made at all. Instead, the best available fit from a range of stock sizes is supplied, at least in hospital. The result is that a really good fit is unusual. But a good fit is essential, and must be insisted on.

THE CHOICE BETWEEN INJECTION AND SURGERY

The choice of definitive treatment for varicose veins thus rests between sclerotherapy and surgery. The aim of both is the permanent ablation of irreparably damaged venous channels, and to hold either method to be in all circumstances the better seems to us unwarranted. There was a time when even the most trivial of surgery was hazardous, and the results of varicose-vein surgery were, to say the least, unpredictable. Clinicians naturally seized on treatment by injection as a promising and preferable alternative. Even today there are still those who compare their results after injection with those of ill-chosen and ineptly-performed operation, in order to 'prove' the superiority of treatment by their method. However, most phlebologists now accept that both methods have their place and proper indications.

Claims have been made that varicosities will sometimes improve or even disappear spontaneously after key lesions, such as incompetent perforators, have been dealt with by injection. But not everyone can accept that this is more than a rarity, and that the claims had been based on sufficiently critical and unprejudiced observation. For our part, we find it easy to believe that simple dilatation, even early lengthening and tortuosity, may be reversible; but cannot believe that fibrosis, such as always develops before long, could disappear again. It would seem to us, therefore, that once pathological changes in the veins are detectable clinically, obliteration of all altered veins is inevitable.

More important than which method is chosen is that the obliteration should be permanent and sufficiently comprehensive. The best results are surely achieved by an enthusiast, himself applying the methods of his own choice and persisting with them until the patient has a good result. In other hands the two methods are not, in our view, of equal merit, though as surgeons we naturally incline in favour of surgery. We would, however, point out that the results of injection are much more variable and less dependable than those of surgery. Often the temptation will arise to give injection a try first; but this can make later surgery very much more difficult.

Reappearance of a varicosity which is supposed to have been dealt with used to occur quite often in the old days of surgical ligature without excision, and it still occurred quite commonly after the old-fashioned thrombogenic injections; a clot often became recanalized, though this rarely if ever occurs with a properly used sclerosant, which leaves only a microscopic clot. Other reasons for local recurrence are the still-occasionally performed ligature without excision, or the missing of a reduplication of a vein, usually a main vein. With surgical excision real recurrence is impossible. Recurrence of the disease, that is development of varicosity in a vein not previously affected, can occur after either method, though it is, as one might expect, seen in inverse proportion to the radicalness of the treatment. When a vein, hitherto unaffected, becomes involved, there has often been the supervention of some additional new factor such as pregnancy. The patient is likely to have been warned that this might occur, and that fresh treatment might become necessary. The patient does not regard such an eventuality as a failure of the first treatment, and as they often come early for further treatment, a few injections may be all that is required.

The more definite the changes in *main* veins or their immediate tributaries, the more the indications lean towards surgery. The more certain the *non*-involvement of main veins, the more the choice inclines towards sclerotherapy. For multiple superficial varicosities and distended veins distinctly adherent to atrophic and eczematous skin, or embedded in fibrous, scarred subcutaneous tissue, injection treatment is the treatment of choice. On the other hand, saccular, thick-walled and relatively large varicosities, under fairly normal skin, are better treated surgically, wherever they are. We also choose injection when the altered veins are intradermal such as spider veins and some of those described under 'The Postphlebitic Syndrome'. Sclerotherapy is also an important adjunct to surgery, for those diseased veins not readily accessible to the knife, or too small and numerous to justify the extensive dissection that would be required.

If the patient is elderly (say over sixty) this will weigh heavily in favour of injection. The special expertise of the clinician will quite rightly be a big factor. He should obviously prefer to use the method with which he knows *he* can get the best results. Accordingly, many patients will have had the choice largely or wholly made for them by their general practitioner when he decides where to refer his patient. For him there will be many who are obvious candidates for one or the other approach, and what is done for the large middle group probably does not matter all that much, provided whatever is done is done well.

There are also, of course, non-medical considerations that may profoundly influence the choice between sclerotherapy and surgery. For example, the position may be altogether different according to whether or not there is a national health service, according to the availability of beds for varicose-vein surgery, and according to the availability of skilled and experienced surgeons prepared to do the work. A well-run clinic run by an enthusiast is certain to get better results, whichever its main line of approach.

THE TECHNIQUE OF INJECTION TREATMENT FOR VARICOSE VEINS

Early attempts to obliterate varicose veins by injection aimed to cause the contained blood to form a clot which became tethered at the site of injection. Nowadays the object is so to injure the wall of the vein that when the empty vein is pressed flat the two sides become stuck together. (There is a microscopic clot of course.) Thus the old bulky clot is avoided and a more dependable and permanent obliteration is assured.

The suggestion was once made, and often repeated, that sclerosants which found their way into healthy, narrow veins would be washed along too fast to do any damage or promote clotting, while where veins were diseased and dilated, and flow was consequently slow, there the chemicals would take effect. The notion may sound all right, but in practice injections of all sorts take effect only close to where they are injected. However, the fact that obliteration only occurs where the injection is given *is* a good reason for giving up the old prohibition of injecting perforating veins. This used to be avoided for fear of precipitating coagulation or sclerosis in deep veins. Now it is often done, though we would not recommend it to the inexperienced. Any material that did in fact reach the deep vein would get so copiously and quickly diluted that it would not constitute any threat to the deep veins, *always provided one does not exceed the limit dose recommended by the manufacturer.*

The principles that the techniques of injection aim to apply are these. The injection of a relatively small quantity of irritant chemical is made by an empty-vein technique, so that there shall be no dilution of the dose by blood, and so that there shall be no question of formation of an obvious clot of blood. The sclerosant is mixed with a froth of air bubbles, so as to increase its effective volume while avoiding dilution. The total amount of material able to be injected at one session being limited by the toxicity of the material (see maker's instructions), several sessions may be required before adequate obliteration is achieved. Our experience has been that to have the best chance of satisfactory obliteration, compression of the vein must be maintained for four to six weeks.

Materials and instruments

1. Plenty of 2 ml ampoules of a suitable modern sclerosant (as opposed to a thrombogenic agent) should be available, in a range of dilutions, the ampoules being sterilized on the outside by being immersed in Hibitaine solution.
2. Plenty of disposable, gauge 22 needles with plastic shanks.
3. Syringes: 2 and 5 ml. Our own preference is for glass as being better able to be handled with sensitivity.

The patient having been examined thoroughly and carefully, the affected veins are marked and the proposed sites of injection ringed with a fibre-tipped pen (Fig. 35). As well as helping with correct injection, these marks will be most useful in assessing the results in due course.

The patient remains standing or sits on the edge of a couch with the legs hanging down. The site for injection is sterilized with a spray. Four to six needles, where necessary bent to 45° adjacent to their shanks, are inserted at the sites previously selected (Fig 36). If the needles have been correctly placed in the venous lumen, blood will be drawn along them by capillary action, and will be seen through the translucent plastic shanks. The patient then lies down. The surgeon takes the foot by the heel and elevates it, placing the sole on his chest (Fig. 37). Thus the vein is emptied, and the surgeon has both hands free for the injections and subsequent bandaging.

Meanwhile a nurse or assistant has been preparing the injection chosen for the **lowest** site. For small intradermal veins, 1 to 2 mm in diameter,

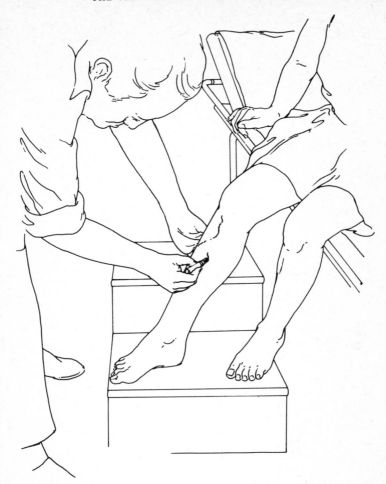

Fig. 35. With the patient standing or sitting every vein requiring injection is marked.

0·5 to 1·5 per cent solution of sclerosant is used, and the 1 ml of injection contains a high proportion of froth. The bubbles are introduced by loosening the needle on the syringe. By adjusting the fit of the needle it is found quite easy to determine the amount of froth and the size of air bubbles admitted as the solution is drawn into the syringe. For larger varicosities, with veins 2 to 4 mm in diameter, 1·5 to 3 per cent solution is chosen, moderately mixed with froth. For varicosities over 4 mm in diameter, 1 ml of 5 per cent solution with little or no air is used.

After each needle has been injected with the quantity and strength

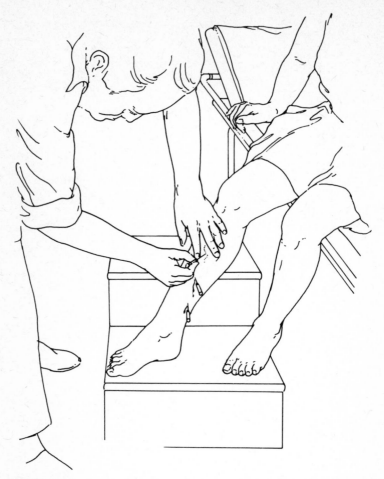

Fig. 36. Needles are inserted at each injection site, also with the patient standing or sitting up on the end of a couch.

selected by the surgeon, the needle is withdrawn. The area is then sprayed and made sticky with Nobecutane. The whole vein is compressed by laying on it a tightly-rolled 10 × 10 cm gauze swab, and fixing it in place with two or three turns of crêpe bandage.

After the last injection and obliteration, the whole leg is carefully bandaged with a firm crêpe bandage, from toes to groin (Fig. 38). Before the patient stands up a much stronger elastic bandage is applied over the crêpe (Fig. 39). This is to be taken off at night, and reapplied before getting out of bed each morning. But the crêpe bandage is to be left

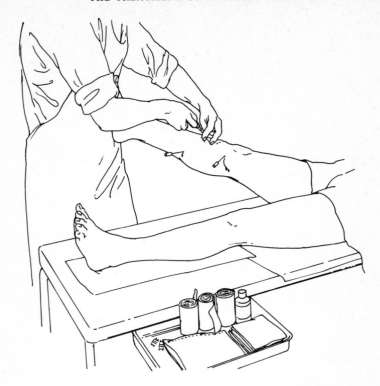

Fig. 37. With the patient lying down and the veins relatively empty, each needle is injected.

undisturbed, if possible for four to six weeks. If it does have to be replaced, this should be done by the original operator. The foot should be raised at least 45 cm (18 in.) and **kept there** while the crêpe bandage is taken off and reapplied securely.

The patient reports for first reassessment with the bandage still on. Any injections that have failed are then repeated. Subsequently the patient should be seen for review and re-injection as necessary at least every 24 months.

Sometimes a segment that has been injected is found not to have been properly obliterated, even though under what seems to have been an adequate dressing. Instead the segment has become filled with black fluid a little reminiscent of a thrombosed external pile. The condition is apt to be painful. It should be treated in exactly the same way by incision and emptying, as described for varico-phlebitis.

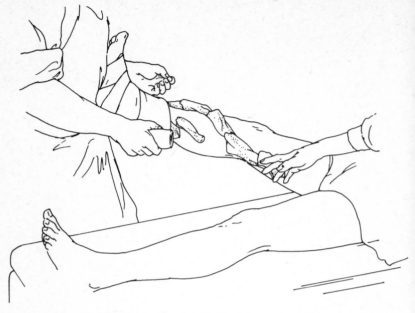

Fig. 38. A crêpe bandage is applied over the dressings.

Complications of sclerotherapy

Deep venus thrombosis

This has been described, but is very rare. (One of us has seen a single case.) However, sclerotherapy should be restricted to ambulant patients, and the leg properly bandaged afterwards. The treatment of deep thrombosis is described in a special chapter.

Necrosis of skin

This occurs at the site of injection. The more usual kind results from injection of a strong solution outside the vein; but another kind is said to occur in spite of injection having been correctly placed, and is reported to be associated with capillary necrosis. A small area of necrosis of skin will be encouraged to slough, and the bare area allowed to heal from the edges. A larger area may be skin-grafted, after careful cleaning.

Allergy

Allergic reactions to any of the materials currently in use is virtually unknown. Should an anaphylactic attack occur, it will be treated along the lines described for a similar attack due to sensitivity to the materials used during phlebography or lymphography (q.v.).

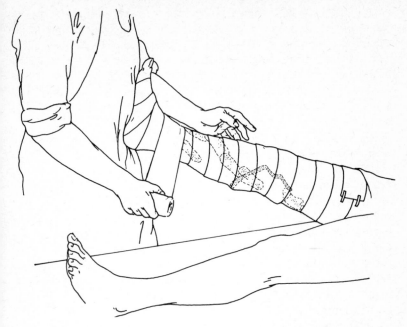

Fig. 39. A strong elastic bandage is applied over the crêpe bandage.

Fainting

Relatively common is ordinary fainting. This is also associated with pallor and low blood pressure. It requires no treatment. If in doubt, assume the attack to be anaphylactic; for no harm will come from resuscitation in an ordinary faint.

SURGERY FOR VARICOSE VEINS

Few surgeons are prepared to take much interest in a field of surgery that they feel to be inexacting as well as unrewarding. All too often varicose-vein surgery in hospital is put to the end of the list, to be relegated to the least experienced member of the team, who scrambles through the operations thinking only of the time when he will no longer have to do them. Yet in no field of surgery is it more true that really good results demand skill, judgement and meticulous attention to detail, as well as a detailed knowledge of local anatomy.

The concept of aetiology on which much current surgical practice for varicose veins is based is this. The most important lesion is incompetence of perforating veins, particularly those on the medial side and above the ankle. These, it is held, allow the very high pressures normally occurring transitorily in deep veins during exercise, to be communicated to the ill-supported superficial veins. It is argued, therefore, that these communications between the superficial and deep venous systems should be severed. On the other hand others have argued that it is irrational to remove any superficial veins at all in a patient who has developed superficial varicose veins on a basis of deep venous obstruction. This notion has been proved quite wrong in practice.

No evidence of inadequacy of drainage into deep veins is ever seen after radical excisions of main superficial veins as well as all dilated perforating veins, and signs appear to be improved in proportion to the radicalness of the excisions.

Probably none would question the need to eradicate segments of vein containing incompetent valves. But there is also such a thing as functional incompetence. Many times we have seen varicosities with a cough impulse or other evidence of potential retrograde flow, yet to our surprise, no evidence of anatomical abnormality of the relevant valve has been visible after its surgical removal. We are bound to judge, therefore, that, just as anatomically normal valves can behave as though incompetent, so apparently competent valves may not in fact always be so. This could account for the also frequent occurrence of varicosities with apparently normally functioning valves above.

There are more valve-like mechanisms in the venous system than the obvious cusped ones, and these too become incompetent, in fact possibly more regularly so, in the condition of varicose veins than the more widely recognized cusped valves. In a normal venous system tributaries ordinarily enter larger veins obliquely. Where they do so a sort of flap valve is formed. In fact, in a normal system, two veins which meet cannot be injected simultaneously from below their junction, for the flow from one closes the mouth of the other. In varicose veins not only are the junctions above a certain size more numerous, also the junctions are nearer to a right angle, and the flap-valve function appears to have been lost. This would imply that any retrograde flow that took place would tend to be more extensive, as well as involving a much larger volume of blood.

Our own view, and we believe it has been proved right in practice, is that a vein which has become **varicose** is doing more harm than good, and always needs to be got rid of.

In the great majority of cases we find that we have to:

1. Strip the great saphenous vein and usually the short saphenous vein as well;

2. Ligature all incompetent or dilated perforating veins;
3. Ablate all altered tributaries as radically as possible.

This may involve attending to more veins than are obviously abnormal clinically. Veins that should be especially examined or which may be found to be abnormal only on such special examination are those participating in what we have called a 'pathological circuit'. When a valve has become incompetent and a vein is the site of retrograde flow, the blood ultimately finds its way into the deep system by an alternative route. The whole of this route tends to become dilated and, in the end, varicose. If any part of this route is left it is apt soon to become part of a new pathological circuit, and the disease will have recurred. We therefore recommend that the whole of every pathological circuit should be identified. This is easiest done by **palpation** in the standing patient. Its total excision is usually found to be indicated.

Clinically it is seldom the main saphenous veins that are obviously varicose, but far more often some of their largest tributaries. It *is* the main veins that are most regularly involved at microscopy. Moreover, evidence of disease is more often than not present to some extent throughout the whole length of the saphenous vein. This is why stripping out of both saphenous veins, or at least the long saphenous is nearly always indicated as part of the operation.

We do not recommend the ligature of perforating veins that are not dilated for, in our experience, those that are not dilated and are left, seldom become dilated later.

Problems arising before operation

Questions to be answered before planning a surgical policy for varicose veins, or before undertaking operation in a particular case.

1. Contraindications

The only contraindication, or factor calling for a modification of approach, is arterial disease. It is well known, of course, that whereas elevation greatly benefits venous disease, it makes the signs and symptoms of arterial disease worse. This is commonly thought to be because dependency eases the flow of arterial blood to the feet, because of the assistance given by gravity. This is mistaken. It does happen to be true that dependency improves arterial supply, but not for the reason imagined. Because the vascular system is a circuit or syphon, the extra impetus given to arterial blood by gravity in the upright position is **exactly matched** by the extra energy requirement to lift venous blood back to the heart. However, when the legs are dependent the extra hydrostatic pressure in all peripheral vessels tends to cause them to dilate. Consequently the resistance that they offer to blood flow through them is disproportionately reduced. Also the fact that capillary pressure in the feet has been greatly elevated, **may** facilitate the transfer of oxygen to the tissues. For the same reason anything else that tends to raise capillary pressure may be advantageous to a patient with arterial disease. For this reason anything which impedes venous drainage must be reduced very gradually and with the utmost caution in arterial disease.

Chronic cardiac disease which is not severe, and which is not uncommon in varicose vein subjects, is not a contraindication to operation. Indeed, patients often profit cardiologically from operation for the venous condition.

2. Prevention of infection by pre-operative antibiotics

On no account should prophylactic antibiotics be allowed to become a substitute for proper pre-operative preparation of the skin. It is not our own practice to use prophylactic antibiotics routinely in surgery for uncomplicated varicose veins. But, if deep veins are to be exposed or handled, or the patient's resistance is for any reason below par, we have no hesitation in prescribing an antibiotic.

3. Should the short saphenous vein be stripped routinely, as well as the long?

Whenever the disease is at all widespread it should. Only when varicosity has remained strictly localized to the medial aspect of the leg for many years, and there are no dilated veins around the lateral malleolus and no palpable short saphenous, may the step be omitted.

4. Is local excision of varicosities alone (without stripping of great saphenous veins) ever justified?

It is justified in patients with no family history of more generalized disease and with isolated varicosities without involvement of either saphenous vein. These are rare, but are occasionally seen, in the popliteal region or on the back or the outer side of the thigh. They always partly drain direct into a local perforating vein, and this must be found and ligated as an essential part of the treatment.

5. When an ankle perforator is to be ligated, should this be done subfascially?

As already indicated we do not practise the routine ligature of all perforators whether or not incompetent and dilated. We would agree, however, that when ankle perforators are incompetent (as shown by their size) it is particularly important that their ligature should not be omitted. We do not accept, however, that this should always be done subfascially, for when these veins are dilated they are easily located through a small local incision. In our view those that are not dilated should be left alone.

6. Can the short saphenous vein be excised from a medial subfascial incision (Cockett's incision)?

We have attempted this in some cases in which such an incision happened already to have been made, but will not do it again. The end of the short saphenous vein cannot be reached and the results of leaving these ends are unsatisfactory.

7. Combined surgery and injection

Often much time can be saved by treating some of the disordered veins by injection, even though the main problem is being dealt with surgically. Some surgeons have to avoid the combination because of having different policies about ambulation after surgery and after injection. Believing in early ambulation after either, we have no such problem. Our practice has been to inject all spider or other intradermal veins at the end of the operation before the dressings are applied. Larger tributaries are excised wherever practicable, and if it is decided to leave any for injection, this is done 2 or 3 weeks later, when any post-operative oedema and bruising have completely settled.

8. What are the risks of thrombosis after operation in superficial veins that have not been removed?

Surprisingly enough, the risk is practically nil. This could be because of the increased fibrinolytic activity known to be present in veins in patients with 'chronic venous insufficiency'.

9. Post-operative deep thrombosis after venous surgery

We have been struck with the fact that deep thrombosis does not seem to occur after venous surgery. We attribute this to early ambulation after operation and to the use of Flowtron leggings wherever special difficulties have arisen.

10. Enlarged veins on the dorsum of the foot

Not infrequently, a patient asks the surgeon to include excision of dilated veins on the dorsum of the foot, in an operation for varicose veins. The reason is nearly always purely cosmetic, and must be judged accordingly. If the veins are excised at all, the excision must be taken right up to the perforating veins which communicate with the deep plantar arch. Otherwise, the stumps are apt to thrombose. Stripping in this area is best avoided as it commonly results in a big haematoma.

11. Vulval varicosities

These are quite different in character from varicosities in the leg, being much thinner walled. Excision is only possible through a number of incisions in the labia majora. Adequate compression is impossible and large haematomas are inevitable. Fortunately, very good results follow injections.

THE OPERATION FOR UNCOMPLICATED VARICOSE VEINS

The night before operation the whole operation area from waist to toes is shaved with an electric razor, and the patient takes a bath. On the morning of the operation he scrubs the area for ten minutes, under a shower. He then visits the surgeon.

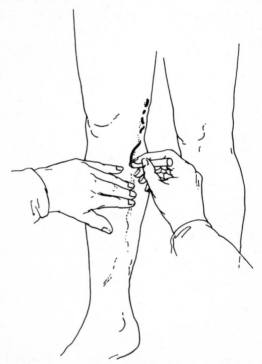

Fig. 40. Every vein requiring attention is marked.

After re-examining the patient the surgeon marks every vein that is to be excised or injected, with a felt-tipped pen, with the patient standing or sitting upright (Fig. 40). Often more veins require to be excised than is obvious clinically, though abnormality is always *palpable* when the examiner knows where to seek, and may be apparent enough on surgical exposure. The vessels involved will be those taking part in what might be called a 'pathological circuit'. For best and most lasting results, the whole of every pathological circuit usually needs to be ablated.

There is little chance that adequate excisions will be done when the surgeon sees the patient for the first time on the operating table. In fact for best results it is imperative that the surgeon should do the marking himself.

Anaesthesia

In some parts of the world the surgeon may have to, or may choose to give his own anaesthetic. In such a case the obvious choice is a low spinal. Because it is safest as well as being technically the easiest to use, we recommend **Pantocain for spinal anaesthesia**. The headache that used to plague patients after spinal anaesthesia was almost certainly due to leakage of cerebro-spinal fluid through an over-large needle puncture; for it has been virtually eliminated by using a really fine, gauge 22 needle. Since the level of the splanchnic nerves is not reached by the anaesthetic, no hypotension results.

Instruments and materials

Sponge-holding forceps.
One 2 ml glass syringe.
Two gauge 19 or 21 needles.
One ampoule of Pantocain powder, sterilized on the outside.
One ampoule of Pantocain Racedrin.
One 22 gauge spinal needle.
File for ampoules.
Towels, swabs, towel clips, etc.

Technique of anaesthesia

Pantocain for spinal anaesthesia is put up by Hoechst as ampoules of dry powder for mixing with the patient's own cerebro-spinal fluid. With each ampoule of powder there is another containing 1 ml of Pantocain solution for local anaesthesia, mixed with a dose of Racedrin, a peripheral vasoconstrictor (to stabilize the blood pressure). Pantocain, when given as a spinal, is all taken up by the tissues locally, and no matter what position the patient subsequently assumes, there is no danger of segments higher than those intended being affected.

The patient lies in the right lateral position with spine fully flexed and with head and knees supported by a nurse.

The skin is prepared and towelled up, exposing L3 and L4.

The injection is to be made between the spinous processes of these vertibrae, and this site is anaesthetized, using one of the **gauge 21 needles** and the solution supplied. The special introducer for the spinal needle may be dispensed with, for it is found that by having used the slightly larger needle for the local anaesthetic, it is quite easy to introduce the gauge 22 spinal needle through the same hole.

After the spinal needle has been located in the spinal canal, 2 ml of C.S.F. is withdrawn with the glass syringe. This is blown into the Pantocain powder. After this has dissolved, the solution is drawn up into the syringe, **using the other (clean) gauge 21 needle**. It is then returned into the spinal canal. The skin puncture is dressed and the patient is put on his back on the operating table.

Instruments for the operation

1. 12 heavy, non-toothed curved 14 cm artery forceps.
2. 1 Moynihan artery forceps, curved serrated jaws—$5\frac{3}{4}$ in. (15 cm).
3. 4 light, curved, non-toothed 10 cm artery forceps.
4. Toothed, insulated dissecting forceps.
5. Non-toothed dissecting forceps.
6. Double-ended retractors: Parkers 7 in. (17·5 cm), Czerny's $6\frac{3}{4}$ in. (17 cm), or Roux 12 cm.
7. 2 McIndoe double-hook skin retractors.
8. 1 Kilner (cat's-paw) retractor.
9. 1 Metzenbaum 14 cm curved dissecting scissors.
10. 1 Mayo straight scissors.
11. No. 15 scalpel blades and holder.
12. 1 Nabatoff stripper (with interchangeable acorns) 6, 9, 12, and 15 mm and cylindrical probe clips.
13. 2 accessory strippers with small, fixed heads.
14. 1 Gillies needle holder.
15. 3 packets of 000 silk for skin.
16. 1 packet 000 chromic catgut.
17. 1 packet of 00 chromic catgut.
18. 3 dozen 8 × 8 cm swabs.
19. Sterile crêpe bandage.
20. 2 abdominal packs.
21. Towels, swabs, towel clips, etc.

Reserve pack No. 1

In a separate sterile pack, for emergencies only:

1. Metzenbaum scissors.
2. Mayo scissors.
3. Nabatoff stripper.

Reserve pack No. 2

Another special reserve pack is kept for dealing with accidental injury demanding repair of a major blood vessel:

1. Three bull-dog clamps.
2. Special arterial atraumatic threaded needles.
3. Suitable needle holder.
4. Fine-toothed dissecting forceps.

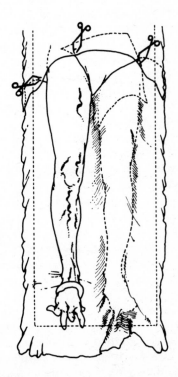

Fig. 41. The towelling-up is complete.

Skin preparation and towelling up

The foot is held by the toes, and the hip flexed and abducted amply. Skin preparation should be conducted into the abdomen, up to the gluteal fold above, and down to the base of the toes. A small towel covers the pubes. A larger waterproof paper sheet, covered with an ordinary one, passes under the leg to be operated upon, and over the other. Finally another large sheet covers the rest of the patient (Fig. 41). Thus only three towel clips are used. A sterile glove is put over the toes.

Stripping the long saphenous vein

A 2 cm skin incision is made below and in front of the medial malleolus, as shown in Fig. 42. The saphenous vein is exposed by *blunt* dissection with artery forceps, delivered into the wound, and divided between artery forceps. Each clamp is picked up in turn, and with its help, all tributaries entering near the end of the vein are isolated, and ligated, or coagulated, as far into the wound as possible. Particularly important, and at the same time easy to miss or somewhat inaccessible, are the submalleolar perforating veins. These must be tied as nearly flush as possible with the posterior tibial vein, and all branches or tributaries must be similarly dealt with. This may require small additional incisions below that just described. The stripper is introduced and fed up to the groin. The small head is attached (Fig. 43).

A 4 to 5 cm oblique incision is made 1 cm below the inguinal crease, starting laterally over the femoral pulse (Fig 44). In an obese patient this incision may need to be a cm longer at each end. The incision is carried down to and just through the very thin superficial layer of the fascia lata. The fat beneath the fascia is parted by **blunt** dissection until the saphenous vein is recognized by its blue colour. The vein is then fully exposed by **pushing** the fat aside (Fig. 45). **This must be done in the correct tissue plane.** Immediately outside the adventitia of the vein there is a sheath of fascia which is particularly easy to separate from the adventitia.

The main trunk of the saphenous vein is now divided between clamps about 3 cm from its termination (Fig. 46). Further **blunt** dissection exposes the termination of the long saphenous in the common femoral vein, and displays all of the group of tributaries that pass through the fossa ovalis, blunt dissection being always exactly in the correct tissue plane. The tributaries must always be dissected **outward** from the main vein. (In fact, following a tributary in order to find the main vein is a

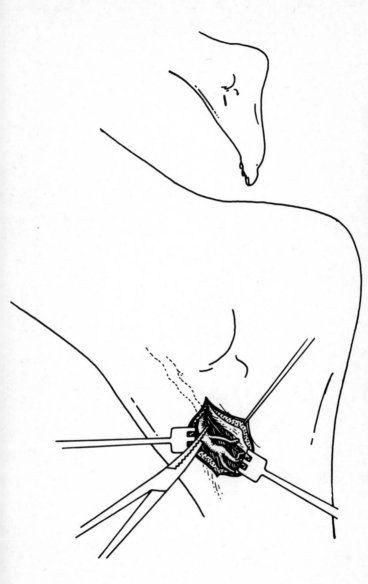

Fig. 42. The great saphenous vein is exposed through an incision in front of the medial malleolus, as shown.

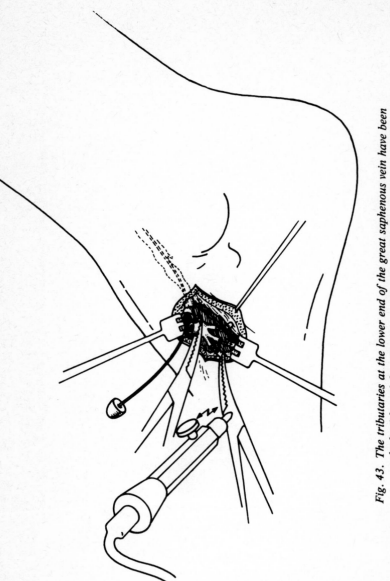

Fig. 43. The tributaries at the lower end of the great saphenous vein have been dealt with, and the stripper introduced and fed up to the groin. The small stripper head has been attached.

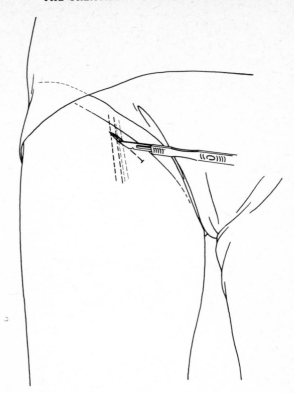

Fig. 44. An incision is made in the groin, as shown.

common preliminary to injury to the main vein.) Each tributary is divided between clamps, the end going to the wound being immediately tied with 000 chromic catgut, and the clamp on the end going to the saphenous vein being put with the others and the clamp on the stump of the great saphenous. The femoral vein is now exposed, the great saphenous doubly ligated with 00 chromic catgut, flush with the common femoral vein.

The stripper is now delivered through the top end of the great saphenous vein. The large stripper head is attached at the top end (Fig. 47). To prevent bleeding coming from the many still intact tributaries, both ends of the saphenous vein are tied round the stripper. By pulling from the ankle end, the trunk is now stripped **down as far as the knee**. This is done with care, so that the extra resistance of a large tributary can be sensed before the tributary is avulsed. If one is felt, a separate incision may then be made, the tributary found, and divided between ligatures

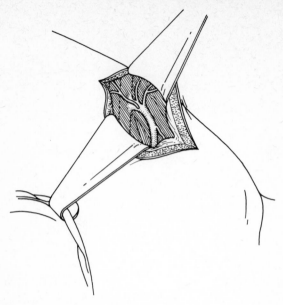

Fig. 45. The great saphenous vein has been exposed. The near retractor hooks conveniently on to the surgeon's waist-tape.

before stripping proceeds any further. Near the knee two or three large tributaries are always found, so the stripping is always stopped at this point. An incision is made on to the stripper head, at the level of the popliteal crease or a little below (Fig. 49).

A smaller head is already attached to the **lower** end of the instrument. From the knee the distal part of the vein is stripped upwards to the knee (Fig. 53). The whole of the vein is now on the stripper. The whole thing may be used to draw any remaining tributaries at this level into the wound, where they are ligated and divided. The same manœuvre to spot and separately divide any larger tributary as described for the thigh is used again for the lower leg. Thus haemorrhage is reduced to a minimum. Bleeding from smaller vessels that have been avulsed is controlled by maintaining firm pressure with the flats of both hands to the tunnel from which the main vein has been stripped, for 5 minutes.

Ligature of perforating veins and excision of varicosities

Mostly these are dealt with in the course of the above operation. Any remaining will require separate incisions.

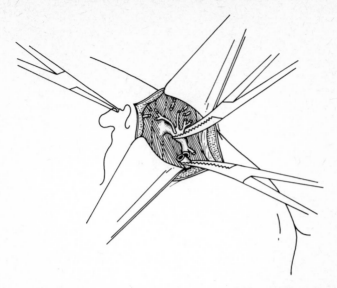

Fig. 46. The tributaries near the end of the great saphenous vein have been dealt with and the great saphenous itself clamped about 3 cm from its termination and severed.

First the perforating veins previously marked with ink circles are displayed superficial to the deep fascia and tied. Then the remaining marked varicosities are excised through as few small incisions as possible, each following Langer's lines, no more than 1 to 1·5 cm long, and 3 to 15 cm apart, according to the tortuosity and fragility of the vein. It is usually possible to dissect each varicosity a long way under the skin by blunt dissection with dissecting forceps and with the help of the double hook retractor. If both ends of a vein are torn off, the central part must not be left, but if the marking has been good it is usually easily found and removed through an additional incision. Longer tributaries with a relatively straight course may be stripped with the small stripper.

Stripping of the short saphenous vein

With the patient still on his back, the knee is flexed to 90° so that the sole of the foot rests on the operating table (Fig. 59).

A 1 to 1·5 cm incision is made below the lateral malleolus (Fig. 54). The lesser saphenous vein is isolated, clamped and ligated. Nabatoff's stripper is introduced at the ankle and fed up the short saphenous vein until it can be felt in the popliteal fossa (Fig. 55).

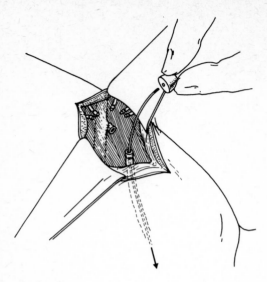

*Fig. 47. The stump of the great saphenous has been tied off, flush with the
femoral vein. The stripper has been delivered from its lower end, and
the larger head is being attached.*

A 2 to 2·5 cm transverse incision is made in or just below the popliteal
crease (Fig. 56). The vein may be identified by inserting a finger under the
fascia, and delivered into the wound (Fig. 57). It is doubly clamped and
divided. By gentle traction on its clamp, the stump may be drawn into the
wound. Often it has a single fine tributary needing attention. The lesser
saphenous is then ligated 2 or 3 cm from its termination. The short
saphenous vein enters the popliteal vein at an acute angle. It has no other
tributaries near this point.

The flap-valve mechanism of the lesser saphenous vein is particularly
well developed. In fact, if it is divided 2 or 3 cm below its termination and
left open, often no retrograde bleeding occurs. Accordingly there is not
the same need to tie the short saphenous flush with the popliteal as there
was to tie the long saphenous flush with the common femoral. The lesser
saphenous is most easily stripped with the surgeon seated, still on the
lateral side of the leg.

When the short saphenous vein has an atypical course, particularly
unusually high or low termination, this is usually recognized with the
stripper, and an ad hoc adjustment to technique made.

The whole leg is now reviewed to make sure that no veins or pieces of
vein have been left behind or not dealt with. If blood is still escaping from

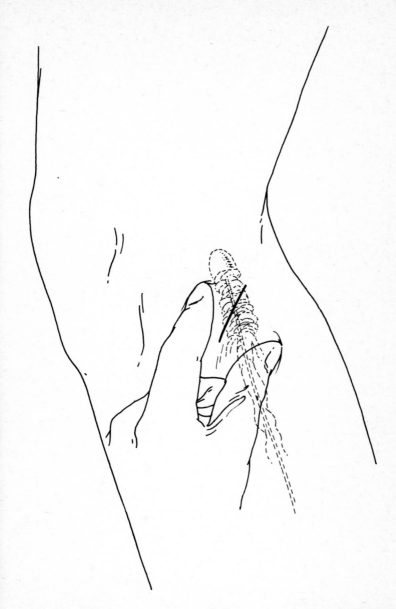

Fig. 48. The great saphenous has been stripped down from the groin to the knee, by pulling from the ankle. The stripper head is being identified through the skin.

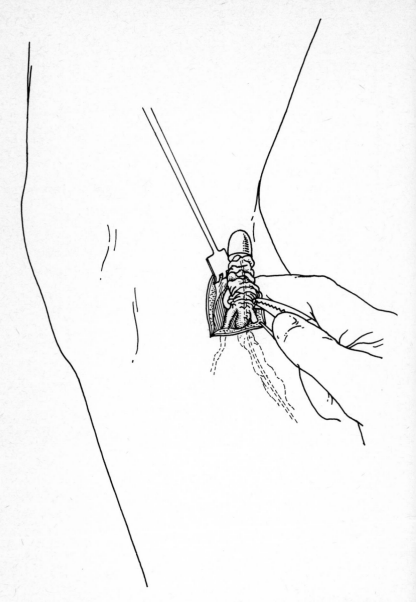

Fig. 49. *The incision has been made as indicated in the last figure. The stripper head with the stripped upper part of the great saphenous vein delivered.*

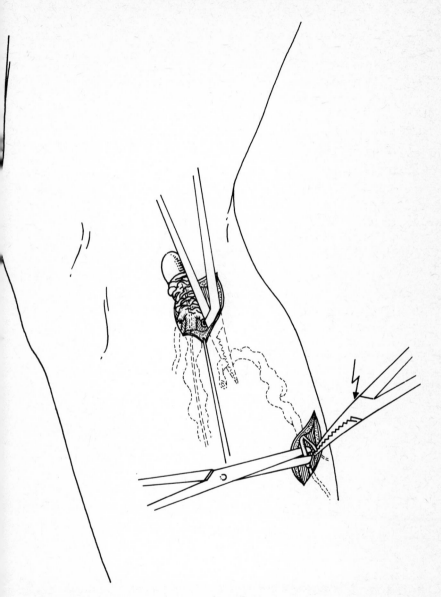

Fig. 50. *A local tributary is being dealt with through a separate incision, by diathermy at its distal end.*

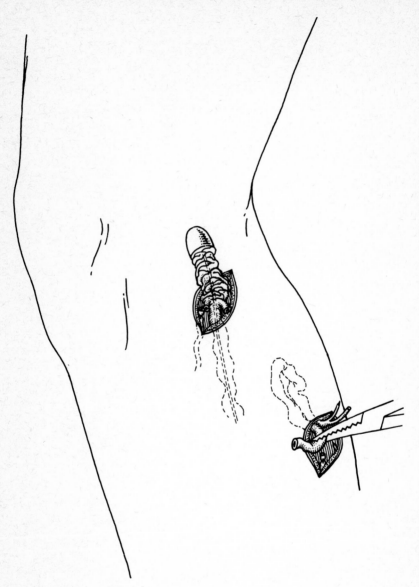

Fig. 51. After dissection, and ligature at its central end, this tributary is being delivered for removal retrogradely.

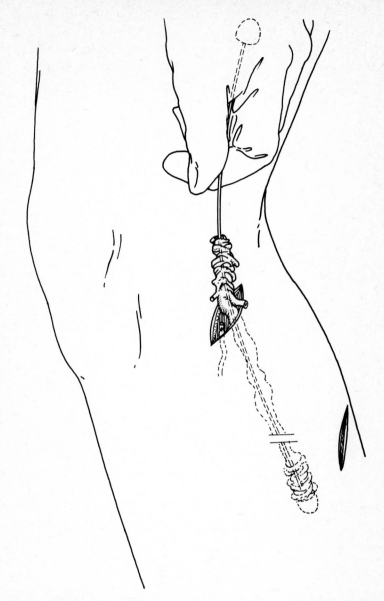

Fig. 52. *The lower part of the great saphenous is being stripped up to the knee. This is done from the lateral side.*

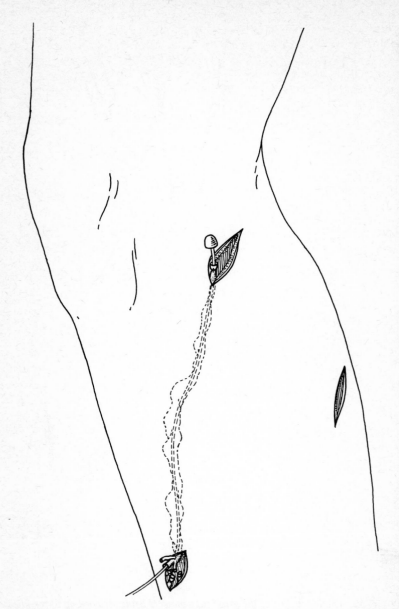

*Fig. 53. Another tributary, being relatively straight, is being dealt with by
stripping retrogradely with the small stripper.*

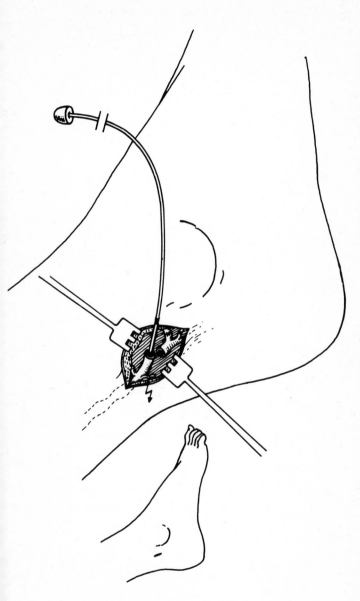

Fig. 54. The lesser saphenous vein has been exposed through an incision behind the lateral malleolus, as shown. Its local tributaries have been dealt with and the main vein has been divided. The stripper has been introduced and fed up to the popliteal fossa. The small head has been attached.

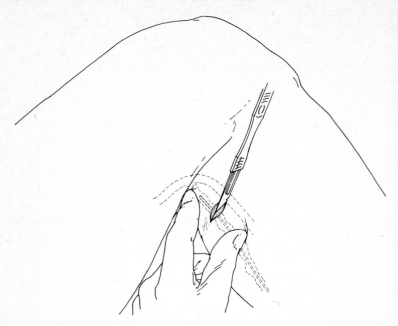

Fig. 55. The shaft of the stripper can be felt through the skin.

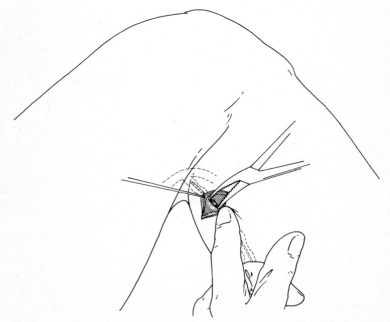

Fig. 56. The lesser saphenous vein is being exposed by blunt dissection.

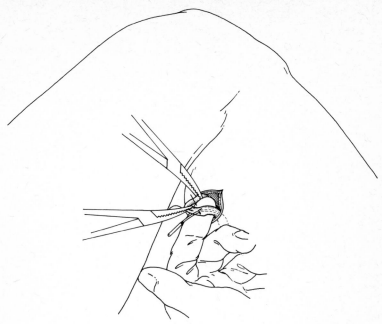

Fig. 57. The lesser saphenous vein is isolated and mobilized with the finger.

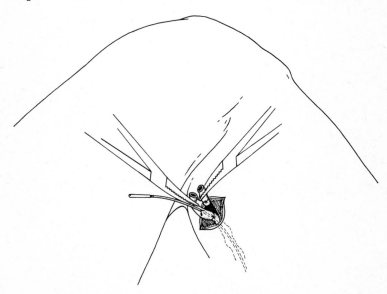

Fig. 58. The lesser saphenous has been divided and its stump entering the popliteal ligated. The stripper shaft has been delivered through the lower part.

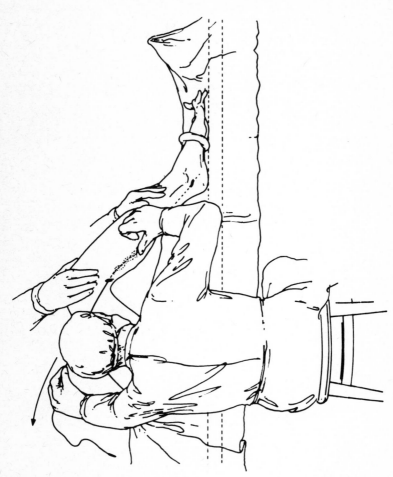

Fig. 59. *The lesser saphenous vein is being stripped. This is most easily done with the surgeon sitting. While one hand pulls on the stripper, the other eases the head along through the skin.*

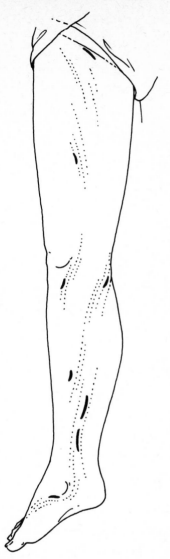

Fig. 60. To illustrate the large number of small incisions usually necessary.

the tunnel in spite of prolonged manual pressure, an abdominal pack is tightly rolled and bound over the tunnel with ordinary cotton bandage.

Elsewhere continued bleeding, if not visible as such, may show itself instead by the bulging of haematoma formation. All blood clots are expressed and all wounds, including the inguinal one, closed in one layer

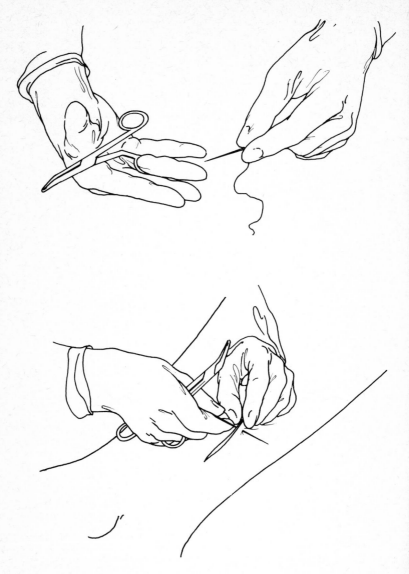

Fig. 61. How to hold a Gillies combined scissors and needle holder (only the scissors part is used when sewing skin with a straight needle). This is much quicker than the usual Continental method of sewing skin with a curved needle held in a holder, which is important in an operation involving a great many small incisions.

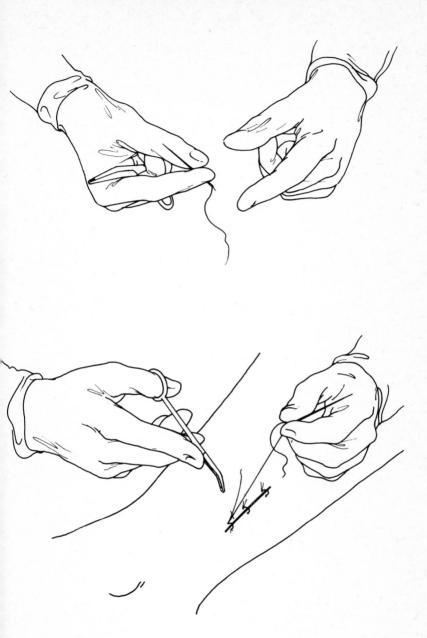

with 0000 or 00000 silk, using a straight needle (Fig. 61). All wounds are dressed and the limb firmly bandaged from toes to groin. The groin wound is above the bandage, and its dressing is fixed separately with Elastoplast (Fig. 62).

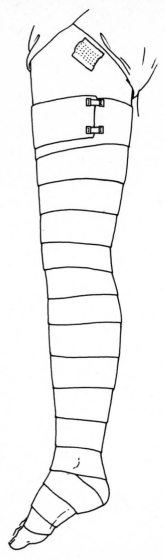

Fig. 62. After the leg has been dressed and bandaged, the groin has to be dressed separately, and the dressing fixed with adhesive strapping.

Post-operative care

The foot of the patient's bed is raised 15 to 20 cm for 24 hours. There should be no pain or discomfort, no pyrexia and no swelling of the toes. The patient is allowed up and encouraged to walk as soon as he has recovered from the anaesthetic (16 to 24 hours). The bandage is left undisturbed for 5 days. The wounds are inspected on the fifth day, when most or all the sutures may be ready for removal. Where necessary, tension on wound edges may be relieved with Steri-strip. According to how much oedema was present before operation, light or heavier dressings are applied. (Below the knee tubigrip may be used.) These are left for a further 10 to 14 days. Any intradermal varices that have been left for injection are dealt with, and the patient is discharged, to attend the out-patients department in 14 days.

Accidents apt to occur during varicose-vein surgery

These may be presumed to occur only with inexperienced operators. But these operations are the ones most often left to beginners, and it is for them that these remarks are intended. Accidents of this sort are predisposed to by incorrectly placed or inadequate incisions, inadequate retraction or lighting, sharp dissection particularly towards instead of away from the saphenous vein, or by ill-chosen ligature material, such as too coarse for small vessels.

Haemorrhage during the operation or soon after

Bleeding is the commonest problem, either during the operation or when the patient first stands. During the operation the source of arterial bleeding is usually easily found. Bleeding of less obvious origin is nearly always venous. In fact it will usually stop after a few minutes of sustained local pressure over a single swab. If it continues the following steps will become necessary. They must be undertaken calmly and deliberately. **On no account must attempts be made to control bleeding by blind stabs with artery forceps**, particularly in areas such as these where serious, irreparable damage may be done. While one hand controls the haemorrhage with well-localized pressure over a minimum of swabs, the other enlarges the incision as necessary. The bleeding point is carefully and deliberately exposed by adequate blunt dissection. If this is found to be in a common femoral vessel, **artery forceps must not be applied even to the side of the vessel**. Instead a special arterial suture mounted on a small, round-bodied, atraumatic needle, is sent for (reserve pack). The tear is now carefully sewn up with minimal narrowing of the vessel.

If the bleeding starts when the patient first stands, it is tempting to lie him down and control the haemorrhage by local pressure. But if one does, and then does nothing more, it will be necessary to leave him lying down for a further several days. This increases the risk of post-operative thrombosis, a risk which is negligible with early ambulation. Accordingly, lying the patient down and applying local pressure must be regarded as no more than a temporary first-aid measure. The patient must then be taken back to the theatre and the wound re-opened and revised.

Haemorrhage from the popliteal wound is less common than from the inguinal one. Bleeding of any note here practically always comes from the popliteal vein. The vein has usually been torn by too vigorous traction on a lesser-saphenous stump. The patient is laid face down with the knee extended, for in this position the lower edge of the popliteal ligament is less in the way than when the knee is flexed. Adequate exposure is more difficult even than in the groin, but must be achieved before such an important repair is attempted. Indeed, before attempting any repair of a major vessel a junior surgeon would do well to make sure no more senior person is available to take the responsibility.

Injury to nerves

Two nerves are particularly at risk during varicose-vein surgery, and no one should embark on operations in this field without being familiar with their anatomy and appearances. The larger is the sural nerve which is a branch of the tibial nerve in the popliteal fossa. It becomes subcutaneous about the middle of the calf where it is joined by the communicating branch from the common peroneal. It then passes down near the lateral edge of the tendo Achillis, close to the short saphenous vein. Behind the lateral malleolus the nerve usually lies behind and medial to the vein. But it is often large enough to be mistaken for the vein. Moreover, it is often surrounded by a bundle of small intercommunicating veins, which bleed when wounded. The sural nerve supplies the lateral side of the foot and a small area on the postero-lateral aspect of the lower part of the leg.

The saphenous nerve is the largest cutaneous branch of the femoral, and arises in the upper part of the thigh. But by the time it reaches the ankle it is smaller than the sural. It passes between the tendons of gracilis and sartorius and then becomes subcutaneous, passing down the medial border of the tibia in company with the long saphenous vein. In the lower third of the leg it divides in two. One branch continues down the margin of the tibia to the ankle. The other stays with the long saphenous vein and supplies the medial side of the foot. At the ankle this nerve is less constant in its relation to the vein, but it is smaller and should seldom cause confusion. In fact this nerve is more often damaged at its bifurcation by the stripper, particularly if too large a head has been used, and stripping is done roughly.

To avoid injury to the saphenous bifurcation one might feel tempted to strip this part of the vein downwards instead of upwards. However, this produces such a bulky mass of vein on the stripper that it constitutes an even greater threat to the nerve.

Post-operative complications

Lymphorrhoea and lymphocoele

Lymphorrhoea is a rare complication usually from one of the incisions in the lower leg, where it arises through division of one of the main lymph trunks. Only the external superficial trunk which runs in company with the short saphenous vein, is regularly at risk. Even so, the complication is rarely seen. This is probably because the lymphatics are so freely interconnected, and they have very substantial regenerative power. Lymphography performed soon after extensive varicose-vein surgery has, in fact, shown several leaks, but always perfectly adequate drainage.

Less rare than lymphorrhoea from the wound is lymphocoele of the inguinal wound. This is believed to be an occasional result of damage to inguinal lymph nodes. A soft, fluctuant swelling results. In our experience these conditions and lymphoedema, which has occasionally accompanied them, have occurred only in the presence of hitherto unsuspected 'hypoplasia' of the lymphatic system. We write the expression in quotes, for the name should imply a congenital condition, and we are by no means convinced that it is.

Lymphorrhoea and lymphocoele both settle in a few days under compressive dressings.

Haematoma of the thigh

If the details of technique advised are followed, bleeding will have been reduced to a minimum and should never constitute a problem. With less meticulous care bleeding can occur and require attention, from tributaries of the great saphenous vein which have been avulsed during stripping. In fact, with full-length stripping, as usually performed, even followed by very firm bandaging, extensive bruising and a certain amount of frank haematoma formation is the rule. If, at the end of the operation, a little bulge somewhere along the tunnel left by stripping denotes haematoma formation, an additional little incision should be made and the bleeding controlled.

Occasionally a firm bar-like haematoma occurs, and is painful and tender. It is due to having missed a saphena duplex. If the duplication of the saphenous has been left and isolated, the contents do not clot. Instead the vein becomes swollen and is found to contain black fluid. After this has been evacuated under local anaesthesia, the symptoms are relieved.

Swelling of the leg

One's first inclination is to suppose the operation to have failed to improve the condition for which it was undertaken, and the oedema to be a venous one. However, swelling of the leg after varicose-vein surgery more often turns out to be due to a latent lymphoedema, and one of the first investigations to make is a lymphogram.

Deep venous thrombosis is a rare complication of varicose-vein surgery. If one is suspected it is managed along the lines described in Chapter 16 and immediate phlebography arranged.

Ugly scar

True keloid scar rarely occurs in the leg except in negroes; but young women not uncommonly get worried about their scars before these have had proper time to settle and turn white. Procrastination is the proper line of management for at least three months. Some have allowed themselves to be persuaded to inject a little hydrocortisone into the scar **intradermally**, but the procedure is very painful.

CHAPTER 15

Treatment of Thrombosis and Thrombophlebitis

THE PREVENTION OF DEEP VENOUS THROMBOSIS

Ideally, effective prophylactic measures would be adopted whenever the slightest extra risk of spontaneous deep thrombosis arose. This would mean with every surgical operation, after childbirth, whenever confined to bed with an illness not incurring operation, and even throughout pregnancy. Even this would not cover the occasional case of 'steamer leg' or of 'air-raid-shelter leg'. However, no less than 2,687 persons were certified as having died from pulmonary embolus in England and Wales during 1971 (the usual cause of fatality when this follows deep-vein thrombosis). Moreover, pulmonary embolism is by no means always fatal and only a small proportion of deep thromboses give rise to a pulmonary embolus. There must therefore be more like 100,000 cases of deep thrombosis occurring in these countries every year. (No wonder there are so many people about who have had this disabling condition.)

Evidently, either no really effective prophylactic measure exists, or it is not being applied nearly so regularly as it should be. Both possibilities are to some extent true. For no drug or measure has yet been shown to be absolutely dependable. But quite simple physical measures can make a remarkable difference to the incidence. Why, then, are they not used more than they are? There are a number of contributory reasons. First, there is a widespread and quite unjustified fatalism about deep thrombosis. This grew up when a case or two occurred as one of the causes of death in nearly every published operation mortality figure, but it was a much less common cause of fatality than some others, and therefore received less attention. Secondly, it was proving one of the most recalcitrant of conditions to prevent. Now there is a danger that the measures advocated will be too simple and uncostly to carry conviction, like the waters of Jordan, and will not be thought worth bothering with.

All that is required is that once every half-hour or even every hour a nurse should see that every patient in bed in a ward, whether surgical, medical, or obstetrical, should quite briefly exercise the legs. Particularly important would be flexion and extension of the ankles and the toes. The flexors and extensors of the thigh and knees, including the buttocks, should be tightened and relaxed, though there would be no need actually to bend the knees or move the hips in any patient for whom such movement was for any reason difficult. At the same time the patient should practice deep breathing. Ambulant patients would meanwhile take a walk round the ward, while doing their breathing exercises. The object is, of course, to prevent the stagnation of blood in the intermuscular veins that is otherwise likely to be occurring. Free exercise of the respiratory pump is probably much the less important, but can do nothing but good.

There is a practical reason why such prophylactic exercises have had to be abandoned by most of those few who have tried them, in spite of their observed success. This is difficulty of persuading the patients to co-operate. Those most at risk, the elderly and the naturally inert, and those who have undergone long operations or had difficult childbirths, are the very ones who most adamantly refuse to move. However, there are two steps that seem to us indicated, and which, to the best of our knowledge, have not been tried. One is to introduce the notion of the importance of occasional movement in bed into nursing training; the other is to organize a regular, say half-hourly, signal during daytime in the wards, coupled with the issue to all patients on admission to hospital of a pamphlet. This should very briefly describe the risk without movement, explain the need for movement, and describe the minimal requirement every time the signal is sounded. (An example that has been used is in the Appendix, no. 10.)

The occasional surgical patient seems particularly convinced that he must lie still after an operation. In addition, surgical patients pass through a period of special immobility, whether unconscious on the operating table or paralysed with a spinal anaesthetic; and the risk is much greater if the operation is a particularly long one. To loss of the calf pump is added loss of the respiratory pump if the abdomen has to be opened. The respiratory pump is not necessarily lost during operations involving thoracotomy because by his manipulations the anaesthetist keeps the diaphragm moving and, so long as the abdomen is not open as well, this affects the blood in abdominal veins. However, throughout this period the blood may be kept moving in the intramuscular veins of the leg with the aid of a Flowtron legging and pulsatile pump. We have tried the effect of these used as well during the post-operative period. The improvement in incidence of post-operative thrombosis has been most gratifying (Pflug, 1965a and b). (See Appendix, no. 9.)

Prophylaxis by drugs

Cumarins or heparin in ordinary therapeutic doses are obviously far too dangerous for pre-operative, or even early post-operative use. The accepted view used to be that heparin in small doses had little effect on the coagulability of the blood. However, for more than ten years Sharnoff and his colleagues have been maintaining that small doses of heparin **subcutaneously** diminished the incidence of pulmonary embolism (Sharnoff, Kass, and Mistica, 1962).

Recently Professor Le Quesne's team at the Middlesex Hospital have re-investigated the effect on the incidence of post-operative deep venous thrombosis of giving heparin subcutaneously. They reported a statistically significant reduction in incidence (Gordon-Smith, Grundy, Le Quesne, Newcombe, and Bramble, 1972). The method is not altogether free from risk.

Platelet adhesiveness can be depressed by certain drugs, notably aspirin and small-molecule Dextran. However, aspirin has failed to affect the incidence of post-operative thrombosis dependably. Small-molecule Dextran during and after operation has seemed more effective, but as it has to be given by intravenous infusion it obviously has limited applicability. So-called anti-thrombotic drugs are popular on the Continent, but are of questionable value and are certainly not to be depended on. The same drugs are also claimed to be anti-oedematous. They do, indeed, reduce oedema, but one of us, after investigating one of the best known, showed its effect to be entirely by inducing diuresis (Pflug, 1973).

All prophylactic treatment for deep thrombosis is at the stage of value assessment, and it is to be hoped that no opportunity will be lost of analysing and reporting results, good or bad. Figures based only on clinical diagnosis or on mortalities are of very little use; for in no field of medicine will simply taking a special interest in and paying more attention to the patients, by itself, be followed by such striking improvement in results. For if it does nothing else, at least it will be bound to lead to earlier diagnosis and treatment.

THE MANAGEMENT OF SUSPECTED
DEEP THROMBOSIS

Early diagnosis and treatment has long been recognized to be one of the most important factors for reducing fatalities from deep thrombosis. A number of sophisticated diagnostic aids are available; but more important than these is sufficiently frequent clinical examination with the diagnosis of deep thrombosis specifically in mind. Detectable swelling may be expected to develop fairly soon in every case of important thrombosis, but earlier and more useful is local tenderness. Most commonly this is found in the centre of the calf; but all the muscles of the legs should be examined, including the thighs, the soles of the feet, and the buttocks. As soon as a serious suspicion of thrombosis arises, 10,000 units of heparin are promptly given intravenously and phlebograms (of both legs) arranged as quickly as possible. This **must** be done as an emergency and not put off till the morning. It can be done by the duty surgeon with the help of a radiographer.

Far the best way of detecting thrombosis in its earliest stages, as well as of following its progress, is by radio-active fibrinogen testing (see Chapter 7). This test has one disadvantage for regular clinical use. It is too sensitive. If every patient with positive findings were to receive a course of heparin, far too many patients would receive this potentially dangerous substance.

Another technical aid of more help in regular screening employs the Doppler ultrasonic apparatus (see Chapter 7). At present this cannot be used below the knee or in obese patients, but with a little experience altered sound over the common femoral veins is readily picked up. Partial obstruction in the femoral veins can be associated with speeding of the stream of blood over a short distance. Popliteal or iliac thrombosis may be expected to slow the stream. Complete obstruction in the femoral vein will completely arrest the flow there, and no Doppler effect at all will be observed. Particularly in mixed types details of change are very difficult to interpret, but so long as any alteration from normal is taken only as an indication for phlebography, this does not matter.

TREATMENT OF DEEP THROMBOSIS

In acute thrombosis or phlebothrombosis, as opposed to thrombo-phlebitis, the clot is not at first adherent to the vein wall, and can be cleared, *provided it is not given time to become organized*. The methods of treatment to be considered include compression, anticoagulents, fibrinolytics, and surgical thrombectomy.

Compression

A compressive bandage is a usual measure, and is popularly argued to work by increasing the velocity of flow in deep veins, as though the deep system was an alternative route from the superficial one for the blood. This is only relatively slightly so. Emptying of the superficial veins by compression may encourage a larger proportion of the blood from epifascial tissues to find its way into the deep veins via the microcirculation. But the clinical effect is minimal, and bandaging should be thought of only as contributing to the patient's comfort.

Anticoagulents

A firm diagnosis of thrombosis is the first step and always requires a phlebogram. The several other methods of investigation available and the technique of phlebography are discussed in Chapter 7. As soon as a clinical diagnosis of deep thrombosis has been made a modest dose of heparin is given, and as soon as the diagnosis is more firmly established the coagulation rate of the blood is brought down properly. It must be kept low for weeks or even months. The anticoagulents available are heparin and the cumarins. All operate by preventing the formation of fibrin. They cannot dissolve fibrin once formed. Though some dissolution may be observed after anticoagulents have been given, this is entirely due to natural fibrinolysis.

Heparin is a naturally-occurring antiprothrombin. It is given intravenously and is effective immediately. It used to be very expensive but currently costs about £1 a dose.

Cumarins prevent the synthesis of prothrombin by being competitive inhibitors of vitamin K. They also hinder the formation of factors VII, IX, and X, all required for the conversion of prothrombin to thrombin. Cumarins begin to take effect about 36 to 48 hours after oral administration.

Though neither heparin nor a cumarin can affect *established* clots, they both prevent further extension or the start of other clots. Clinical experience has also been that they almost eliminate pulmonary embolism. Heparin is much the safer because, as well as being the more predictable as to patient response, also it has much the more dependable and promptly-acting antidote. However, no anticoagulant is entirely free from the risk of promoting haemorrhage. Apart from bleeding into a recent surgical or other wound, or from a recently parturient uterus, the commonest forms of spontaneous haemorrhage are: epistaxis, bruising, haematuria, and gastro-intestinal loss. Apoplexy can occur in an elderly patient.

The cumarin Tromexan ceases to act soon after the last dose, for it leaves the circulation at a rate of about 25 per cent per hour. Warfarin persists much longer, being eliminated at a rate of about 17 per cent per 24 hours. Though in the main conforming to these figures, responses to cumarin vary from patient to patient, and from occasion to occasion in the same patient.

In practice the quick-acting heparin is given at once, and a cumarin given by mouth at the same time, and the heparin has to be maintained for two or three days until the cumarin can take over. Immediately on clinical diagnosis of deep thrombosis, 10,000 units of heparin are given intravenously. The diagnosis is then confirmed by phlebography. If it is so, and heparin is the chosen treatment, an intravenous drip is set up. This consists of 40,000 to 60,000 units of heparin in 4 bottles of 5 per cent glucose solution to be given in 24 hours (16 drops per minute). Approximately this dosage is maintained for 3 to 5 days. The precise dose may be regulated on the basis of the whole-blood clotting time (Lee White), the result being expressed as a percentage of normal, and the aim being to keep it at about 50 per cent of normal. Clinicians very familiar with the use of heparin often cease to feel any need to monitor the dose in this way.

The dose of cumarin is monitored by frequent estimations of prothrombin time (the time taken for a blood sample to clot, after the addition of an excess of Ca ions, and of thromboplastin). This test may not be dispensed with. The time is also expressed as a percentage of normal. The aim is to keep this figure at about 20 per cent of normal. Prothrombin estimations are done daily at first, but as the patient's level of response becomes steadier, they may be done less frequently, ultimately fortnightly for very long-term treatment.

The following are absolute contraindications to the use of cumarins, and make heparin very dangerous: any disease associated with bleeding, such as peptic ulcer, ulcerative colitis, arterial hypertension, detached retina, apoplexy, purpura, and blood dyscrasias. The cumarins should also not be used in pregnancy, and they are avoided in the elderly, in chronic alcoholism, and in unco-operative patients. They may not be given in combination with most of the analgesics (including aspirin, its derivatives), other salicylates, butazolidine, and the oestrins.

Antidotes

The action of heparin may be immediately arrested by giving protamine sulphate intravenously in the correct dosage. Circulating heparin is destroyed in all living tissues by heparinase, at a rate in man of about 25 per cent per hour. What is calculated to be left is neutralized by 10 mg of protamine sulphate per 1,000 units of heparin. Within one hour the patient's reactivity to further heparin should have returned to normal.

The cumarins are antagonized by sufficiently substantial doses of vitamin K. This should be given by mouth. Intramuscular injection is permissible if action must be prompt; but intravenous injection is to be avoided. After vitamin K the action of further cumarin is uncertain. In the main it depends on the dose of K given, but the effect is not constant. It is best not used unless absolutely necessary.

The fibrinolytics

The fibrinolytics are proteinolytic enzymes with a capacity to digest fibrin. They are not able to affect the collagen of organized clot, and do nothing to living tissue. Conversion of fibrin to collagen in a venous clot ordinarily begins in about 48 hours. Fibrinolytics accelerate the conversion of plasminogen to plasmin.

Streptokinase is obtained from streptococci and is antigenic. Anyone who has ever had a streptococcal infection, scarlet fever, a severe sore throat, puerperal fever, lymphangitis, etc., has some anti-streptokinase in his blood. This must first be neutralized before the clot can be assailed. It is possible to estimate the patient's titre of antibody. But the easier and more usual way is to give an adequate loading dose. The initial dose should therefore exceed 25,000 units. (The recommended first dose varies somewhat. There are side-effects from excessive dosage.) As well as its fibrinolytic activity, streptokinase has some anticoagulent action by discouraging platelet aggregation, by digestion of agglutination factor, and by partially inactivating thrombin. Streptokinase may also cause allergic manifestations: fever, rigors, hypotension, and rashes, all preventable by previous injection of 100 mg of hydrocortisone.

Urokinase has exactly the same action as streptokinase, but is neither toxic nor antigenic, and there is almost no circulating antibody. But it is more prone to promote coagulation and is prohibitively expensive. (A day's medication costs between £400 and £700.)

At present no fibrinolytic drug is suitable for use anywhere but at a special centre, equipped and staffed to cope with all the highly sophisticated and time-consuming estimations necessary in the proper monitoring of this treatment.

Thrombectomy

Thrombectomy is a mechanical approach to an essentially bio-chemical problem. Thrombosis, as was explained earlier, is an incident in a continuing disease and there is a strong tendency for the clot to reform. Thrombectomy must, therefore, always be combined with anticoagulent therapy. The earliest day or two after operation are therefore critical. Nevertheless, there are many occasions where it offers a safer and in some ways simpler method of treatment, and others where it is the only method of treatment with any chance of success at all. There is no danger of freeing a thrombus, and then losing it into the circulation, so promoting pulmonary embolism, provided a proper technique is followed, and provided a local or spinal anaesthetic is used, so that the patient may carry out Valsalva's manœuvre when asked, or provided the patient is intubated and the anaesthetist present.

Because the effect of heparin may be instantaneously stopped with protamine sulphate it is safe to use heparin before or after operation, though it is used only with special care in the earliest days after operation. Thrombolytic agents may be used before operation but not after. Cumarins must not be given before surgery.

SUMMARY OF MANAGEMENT OF ACUTE DEEP THROMBOSIS

Medical

1. 10,000 units of heparin intravenously on first suspicion.
2. Phlebograph *as soon as possible and on no account later than 24 hrs.*
3. A. If this shows incomplete obstruction, and not too adherent a thrombus (this often has to be taken as 'not more than 48 hrs have passed since onset'): fibrinolytic therapy, followed by not less than 6 weeks of anticoagulants.
   B. If the phlebograph shows complete obstruction, or more than 48 hrs has passed since the onset: thrombectomy, followed by at least 10 weeks of anticoagulants.

The chances of success with either method depend on the degree of adherence of the thrombus. Some radiologists are able to give an opinion about this.

Though we do not, as some do, regard thrombi more distal than iliac or femoro-popliteal ones as unsuitable for thrombectomy, they are in fact nearly always offered for surgery too late for it to be considered. They are also too late for fibrinolytis. Long-term anticoagulants are recommended, to prevent further extension or the commencement of other thromboses. Otherwise such measures as elastic stockings and intermittent use of the Flowtron legging are all that remain, to be used as indicated.

Post-operative thrombosis

If a suspicion of deep thrombosis arises during the earliest four days after operation, and heparin therefore may not be given, treatment with small-molecule Dextran is indicated. 500 ml of Dextran solution is given in 2 hours, and phlebography proceeded with.

As soon as the diagnosis has been confirmed, thrombectomy is undertaken. This is followed by a small heparin drip, at a rate of 5,000 units per 4 hours. After the first critical 48 hours the dose may be gradually increased. After the beginning of the fifth day full dosage of heparin may be used, subject to the results of whole-blood clotting time estimation. A cumarin is also started on the fifth post-operative day, to take over from the heparin two or three days later. This is maintained for at least 10 weeks.

Thrombosis starting more than four days after operation is treated exactly as in the 'medical' group above.

In pregnancy

Cumarins are strictly avoided on account of the risk to the foetus, for unlike heparin, cumarins can pass through the placenta. Prolonged administration of heparin is obviously impracticable, and the fibrinolytics have not been judged free from risk. However, having been convinced that thrombokinase would carry the lowest risk of available methods of approach, one of us has in fact used it in pregnancy with good results, for many years. Occasion has not arisen to give it in the first trimester.

First the diagnosis is confirmed by phlebography, always being sure that an image intensifier is available, so that the dose of X-rays required may be kept to a minimum. Next the patient's titre of anti-streptokinase is estimated, rather than give what may be an unnecessarily large loading dose. The loading dose is adjusted accordingly. After that streptokinase administration proceeds as described.

Puerperium

The same regime applies as in the post-operative group, the parturient uterus being regarded as an operation wound. Careful charting of blood loss by weighing, is used.

TECHNIQUE OF STREPTOKINASE ADMINISTRATION

1. Under local anaesthesia and through as small an incision as convenient, a vein is isolated in the dorsum of the great toe, as for phlebography (see Technique of phlebography: Chapter 7).

2. A cannula is introduced, if possible, towards the tip of the toe, but if not, proximally, a good 1·5 cm. This is fixed in position with a double length of 0000 chromic catgut. The vein behind the cannula is tied off with a single piece of the same material, of which the ends are left long. This facilitates recovery of the vein if the cannula slips out, as it is so apt to do during nursing procedures.

3. A blood sample is collected for laboratory tests.

4. The venous pressure is recorded both at rest and during activation of the calf pump, for later comparisons.

5. Phlebography is performed, for confirmation of the diagnosis.

6. Hydrocortisone 100 mg is given via the cannula.

7. Flowtron leggings are applied to both legs and a Kidde's tourniquet is put round the thigh on the side to receive the streptokinase, all to be maintained throughout the rest of the treatment with streptokinase. A Kidde's tourniquet is an inflatable bag tourniquet (like a sphygmomanometer) which is fitted to the thigh to direct the blood carrying the streptokinase into deep veins. It is blown up from a cylinder of compressed gas, to a pre-set pressure of 40 mm Hg.

8. Loading dose: 250,000 units of streptokinase in 5 ml of water are mixed with another 100 ml of glucose or saline, as recommended by the manufacturer. This is given in 30 mins.

Further dosage: Subsequently 500,000 units of streptokinase is made up with **500 ml** of solution. This is given as a drip into the cannula over the next **6 hours**. This rate is maintained, subject to the results of the investigations, for not less than 3 days, and not more than 7.

Frequent laboratory testing is essential to control the rate and dosage of streptokinase, and the tests must include thrombin clotting time and euglobulin clot-lysis time on blood samples taken before the start of the treatment, 30 minutes after the end of the loading dose, and subsequently every 24 hours. If possible these tests should also be carried out: plasma fibrinogen, blood platelet count, and haemaglobin estimation. If all these results are properly watched the risk of haemorrhage is reduced to practically nil. Phlebography is also repeated at 24 and 72 hours, for comparison with the radiographs taken before the course of streptokinase was begun.

It is an ascending, dynamic one using 60 ml of 50 per cent Lipiodol, through the infusion cannula, and with a venous tourniquet above the ankle.

Should an antidote become necessary, the usual aminocaproic acid is not so good as a small (half bottle) blood transfusion. Aminocaproic acid is given (100 mg per kg of body weight) only if the transfusion fails to control the situation.

After the termination of the streptokinase treatment, heparin is given at a dose of 40,000 u per 24 hours, for 3 days. Cumarin is started at the same time as the heparin so that it is acting fully by the time the heparin is stopped.

THE TECHNIQUE OF THROMBECTOMY

Anaesthesia. Spinal anaesthesia is often recommended so that the patient may co-operate by performing Valsalva's manœuvre as required. However, if a general is used and the patients intubated, the anaesthetist's manipulations of his bag may be more dependable.

Thrombectomy should not be attempted unless the facilities are available for performing phlebography on the operating table.

The gross appearances of restoration of flow are not enough as an index of successful and complete thrombectomy.

The instruments will be the same as those described for uncomplicated varicose veins in the previous chapter with the addition of O'Shaughnessy's artery forceps curved on the flat with serrated jaws, $8\frac{1}{2}$ in., and a set of Fogarty catheters.

1. A cannula is inserted into a dorsal vein of the great toe as described for phlebography in Chapter 7.

2. A 6–8 cm groin incision is made as described for stripping of the great saphenous vein.

3. The termination of the great saphenous vein in the common femoral vein is dissected.

4. The common femoral **artery** is mobilized and supported by a loop of tape.

5. Four or five cm of the **common femoral vein** with its tributaries, is mobilized and taped at each end of the segment (Fig. 63).

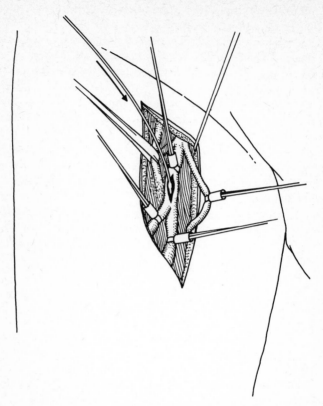

Fig. 63. The great saphenous vein and the femoral artery are being retracted with tapes. The common femoral vein has been opened between the junction of the superficial and deep femorals (to form the common femoral vein) and the termination of the great saphenous vein.

6. If the thrombus is in the deep veins of the lower leg as well, an additional 1·5–2 cm incision is made beneath each malleolus.

7. While the patient is trying to exhale against a closed glottis (Valsalva) and the foot-ward end of the segment of taped common femoral veins is being held closed, the vein is opened. A 1·5 cm longitudinal incision is made just towards the head from the termination of the great saphenous vein. Usually any clot in the common iliac veins is promptly extruded.

8. The iliac veins are checked with a Fogarty catheter. This is an 80 cm gum-elastic catheter with a little balloon at the tip which can be inflated from the proximal end. Sizes 6, 8, and 10 (French) are usually

available, with balloons that can be inflated to 1·5, 2·5 or 4 ml. This is passed well into the vein with its balloon uninflated. The balloon is then blown up until it can be moved along the vein only with firm resistance. The catheter is then withdrawn so loosening and bringing with it any remaining clot.

9. The *proximal* end of the common femoral vein is now held closed with the other tape, and clots encouraged to escape from the main deep veins, by kneading the leg, milking accessible veins and finally, by Fogarty catheter introduced retrogradely.

10. When the posterior tibial vein is obstructed, the sub-malleolar perforator is so dilated that the smallest Fogarty catheter can be introduced through it, into the posterior tibial vein and passed up this anterogradely. Usually the catheter itself is an adequate fit without inflation of its balloon. At the popliteal fossa the balloon of the Fogarty catheter is inflated, and dislodged clot pushed on to the groin, where it is delivered.

If the Fogarty catheter will not pass, an attempt to free the clot with a suitably-sized stripper is made, and the catheter tried again.

11. The leg veins are then flushed through with heparinized saline (5,000 units to 20 ml of saline) from every opening distally up to the groin. All venotomy wounds are closed with 00000 silk on atraumatic needles; a last check of flow being made before each stitch is finally tied.

12. A drip of 7,500 units of heparin in 500 ml of 0·9 per cent (normal) saline is set up, running into the cannula on the great toe.

13. 20–30 minutes later a phlebogram is performed on the operating table. A light tourniquet is applied above the ankle to direct the material into the deep veins and 30 ml of 40 per cent of Hypaque is injected into the great-toe cannula.

If no evidence of thrombi is seen, the skin wounds are closed, and a compressive dressing applied from toes to groin as after stripping of saphenous veins.

On arrival in the ward the foot of the bed is raised 30 cm to reduce venous pressure and dilatation and maintain velocity of flow. Heparin infusion continues at a rate of 35,000 to 40,000 units per 24 hrs for 3 days. Cumarin is given, starting at the same time. The heparin may be reduced on the second and third day, according to the results of the Quick test, and stopped on the fourth day. The cumarin must be continued for at least 6 weeks. Ambulation should begin and be encouraged directly the heparin infusion ceases.

THROMBOPHLEBITIS

Two forms of superficial thrombophlebitis are recognized: thrombophlebitis migrans and varicophlebitis. Both are confined to superficial veins.

Thrombophlebitis migrans

In the first place the treatment is conservative. An elastic bandage is applied and phenyl butazone 200 mg (with meals) given on the first day. Subsequently, a dose of 100 mg per day is maintained for 3 or 4 weeks. If the condition recurs, stripping of the saphenous veins, and excision of all involved tributaries must be considered. In our hands the condition has not recurred again after this treatment. Phlebitis migrans is supposed to precede Buerger's disease, but we have never seen this happen, in any of 23 patients followed from 5–15 years.

Varicophlebitis

Varicophlebitis is commonly feared to be associated with deep venous thrombosis but this is not so, and no special prophylactic measures against deep thrombosis are called for. The essential step, as in thrombosed external pile, is to incise the vein and turn out the tense clot. This may be done under local anaesthesia, though none is necessary in a phlegmatic patient. A No. 11 blade is commonly laid out. This has a tapering shape and is very apt to make a smaller cut in the vein than it does in the skin. Instead a No. 15 blade should be used, held vertically. A small stab incision is made, with the cut in the vein the same length as that in the skin. The whole of the clot is expressed. Thrombolytic ointment or gel is applied and the wound left open. A foam-rubber pad completes the dressing which is left for 10–14 days. Throughout this treatment the patient is ambulant.

CHAPTER 16

Treatment of Postphlebitic Disease and of Chronic Venous Insufficiency

In postphlebitic disease it used to be assumed that, as in arterial disease, loss of carrying capacity was the cause of the changes observed. For it was not appreciated that drainage **efficiency** could be anything but the same as loss of volumetric capacity of the drainage channels. Attempts at cure in postphlebitic cases consisted of various ingenious manœuvres designed to provide a new drainage channel. The obvious choice as 'donor' for such a purpose was the great saphenous vein; for this vessel had already shown itself able to be dispensed with in its usual role. The cross-over plastic of Palma and Espéron (1959) and some other operations, made use of a largely free graft of this vein. It was no surprise that the graft soon became blocked with new thrombus; for after loss of its proper blood supply, at least parts of the vein must die and promote clotting in its contents.

However, thrombosis was more usually blamed on the need to have a venous suture line, which was supposed to initiate the new clot. But suture of a wounded or even transected healthy vein seldom precipitates clotting, and a good result is the rule. Attempts were made to keep the graft patent by making a small anastomosis with an artery (Bryant et al., 1958). These were successful for a time but in our hands always led to re-thrombosis soon after the artery had been disconnected again. One reason for the different behaviour of the graft might be that a patient who has suffered a spontaneous thrombosis still has a chronic disease characterized by a greater-than-normal propensity to form clots. Another might be that once the blood has been persuaded to adopt a different route, it is not all that easy to coax it into yet another.

Meanwhile, other surgeons had turned their attention to the problem of persisting inadequacy of venous drainage after a vein that had been

217

clotted, had become re-canalized. It was pointed out that after re-canalization it was most unlikely that normal function had been restored to the valves. Accordingly, loss of valves was held to have encouraged retrograde flow whenever the pressure gradient had become adverse. (Particularly this would occur when an accessory pump was activated, for, as explained in Chapter 4, these cannot work without first closing an upstream valve. Loss of upstream valves therefore puts an accessory pump out of action. For example, loss of valves near the top end of the femoral and great saphenous veins, would imply that deep inspiration or a Valsalva's manœuvre, would be bound to promote retrograde flow down the great saphenous; and loss of valves in the popliteal vein would imply that blood recently ejected from the calf pump, could flow back in again on calf relaxation.)

It was also held that dividing the femoro-popliteal column of blood in two, would reduce the hydrostatic pressure in veins at the ankle. Accordingly, Gunnar Bauer (1948) introduced ligation of the popliteal vein, and Linton (1938) recommended tying the superficial femoral. One of us used one or other of these operations over 200 times. In a series of 180, the results of combining Bauer's or Linton's operation with routine varicose-vein surgery (as here described) were compared with those of performing varicose-vein surgery alone on another, matched series (Pflug, 1965a and b). No differences could be observed and it was concluded that neither operation had any lasting advantage to offer. It was noticed, however, that the typical bursting pain of old deep thrombosis was nearly always relieved.

The failure of Bauer's and Linton's operations we attribute to these facts. Firstly, neither operation did anything to restore dilatability and contractility to the vein that had been involved; features which we think as vital to proper function of big veins as normality of valves (see Chapter 3). Secondly, we hold that the notion that ligature of a main deep vein would make any difference to hydrostatic pressure in foot veins during forward flow of blood, was mistaken. (It could modify only the effects and extent of retrograde flow.) It could do so indeed, **if the blood had been stationary**, but not in forward-moving blood. For in order to maintain forward flow the pressure in foot veins has to be large enough to overcome a hydrostatic pressure equivalent to the vertical height of the heart, *with or without the ligatures*.

We cannot, therefore, recommend any of the operations designed to replace lost carrying capacity after deep thrombosis. Indeed, we do not believe that this is often seriously impaired. The **immediate** loss we hold to be in efficiency of pumping by the accessory pumps, and no operation yet devised does anything to improve this. Nor can we recommend any of the ligatures for the same reason. We have argued that most of the **late** effects of deep venous thrombosis are due to the secondary dilatations that develop gradually through the years. Once trophic changes have appeared, extensive ablations of dilated superficial veins and perforators, can be depended on much to improve the patient's lot; though they do not cure the basic causative lesion. The long-term results of the operations about to be described are in inverse proportion to the severity of the remaining damage to the deep venous system.

In **chronic venous insufficiency** the disease process is mainly confined to superficial tissues. Deep thrombosis, when it has occurred, has more often been an incidental complication of relatively minor importance. The results of the same operations are, as might have been expected, excellent and lasting.

TECHNIQUE OF OPERATION

The technique of operation is the same, whether the condition is postphlebitic or not. Since the operation is a little different according to whether the skin is loose or of normal tension, or whether it is excessively tight, the descriptions are divided accordingly.

Infection of a wound is very apt to cause marginal necrosis, a complication which commonly occurs when incisions have to be made through trophically damaged skin; even without infection. For this reason it is as well always to start antibiotic treatment on the evening before operation, and continue it for six days afterwards.

Loose skin or skin under normal tension

In most areas an operation identical to that described for varicose veins is carried out; the only difference being that the ablations are likely to be very extensive. On the medial aspect of the lower leg, however, where trophic changes are always most marked, undermining of the skin is largely impossible, and the usual technique of stripping of the great saphenous veins seldom wise. The incisions near the ankle and in the groin are made as described in Chapter 14, and the upper and lower ends of the great saphenous vein dissected out. The stripper is introduced at the lower end, as previously. It is passed upwards cautiously. If it sticks it is withdrawn, reintroduced into the top end of the vein, and another attempt made to pass it retrogradely. If it sticks again it is withdrawn and passed up from below again. This time it is left in situ.

A longitudinal incision is now made in the lower leg. This incision is often serpentine, the aim being to unite all the largest visible or palpably dilated veins. It also passes over the stuck stripper end (Fig. 64). (The origin of these veins is not important; that is, whether they are sections of

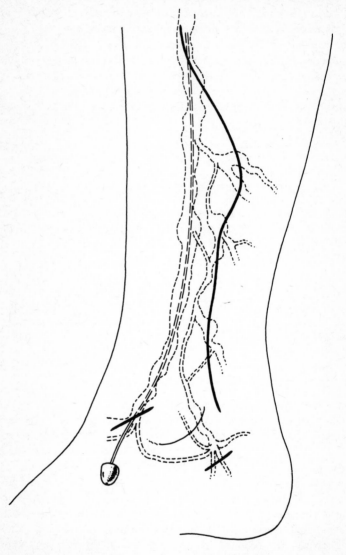

Fig. 64. Redundant skin. The skin incision on the medial aspect of the lower leg crosses as many prominent varicosities as possible.

The incision is closed as a single layer, with interrupted 000 silk, without drainage (Fig. 71).

The short saphenous vein and its tributaries are dealt with as previously described.

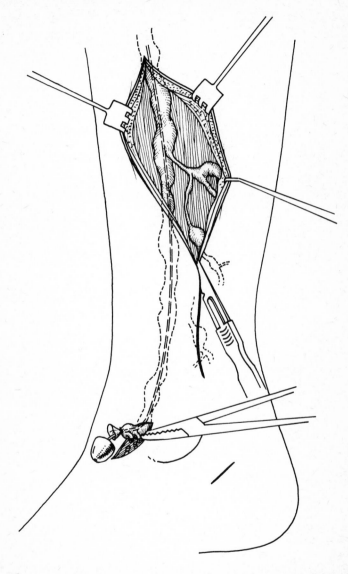

Fig. 65. Redundant skin. All veins are approached from outside the fascia.

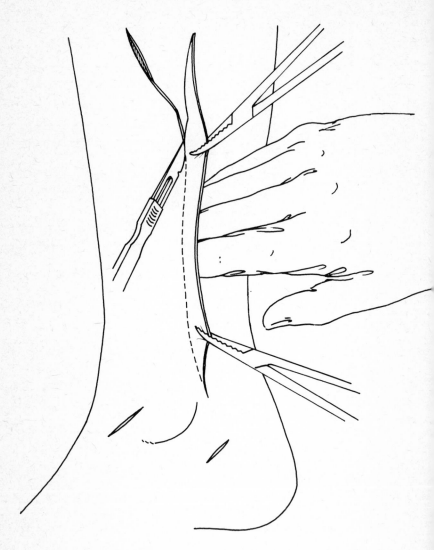

Fig. 66. Excision of redundant skin.

the great saphenous, or its tributaries, or perforator veins.) The intention is to remove these dilated veins as completely as possible, along with the skin to which they are attached. This will be found to have included the worst affected areas of skin. The stuck stripper end is usually easy to free by 'milking' the vein locally, after the direct approach. It can then be passed on to the groin.

Finally, the great saphenous vein is stripped in two halves as previously, the lower half often needing help from outside the vein.

Where the stripper has stuck it can be eased along by a direct approach from outside the vein (Fig. 65). Stripping is done up and down to the knee, as previously.

The short saphenous vein and its tributaries are dealt with as previous described. Finally, the redundant skin is trimmed off (Fig. 66).

Tight skin

The difference lies in the method of making the 'paratibial' incision. The incision is started above in a relatively healthy area, and is carried right through the deep fascia straight away. The incision is not all made at once, but step-by-step, to avoid excessive blood loss (Fig. 67); each segment being rendered as bloodless as possible before proceeding to the next. After the first section two fingers may be introduced under the fascia, and advanced under the next section (Fig. 68). This may then be incised between the two fingers.

Veins of considerable size, having predominantly longitudinal courses, repeatedly cross the line of the incision. Also encountered are smaller tributaries with mainly horizontal courses. These tend to retract into the fibrous tissue. They are coagulated with diathermy when this can be done without burning the skin, bearing in mind the strong propensity to marginal necrosis. Or they may be under-run with a 000 chromic catgut stitch. The perforating veins are best displayed by lifting the deep fascia, when they can be seen beneath the fascia, crossing the subfascial space (Fig. 69). Here they are doubly sutured with 000 chromic catgut passed on an aneurysm needle, and divided between.

Tributaries of the short saphenous vein can be dealt with through short local incisions in the ordinary way, for the skin on the back of the leg is not nearly so bad.

Stripping of the long saphenous vein is carried out as just described, except that if the stripper becomes stuck it can be exposed by an incision through the fascia from **behind it**, after approaching it subfascially (Fig. 70). Any segments that have to be left behind may be treated later by injection.

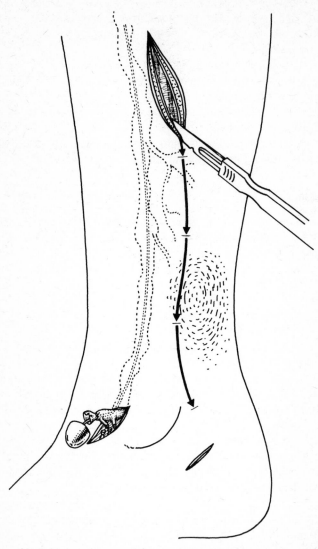

Fig. 67. *The skin incision is carried right through the deep fascia, and is made in three to five steps, so that haemostasis may be obtained after each.*

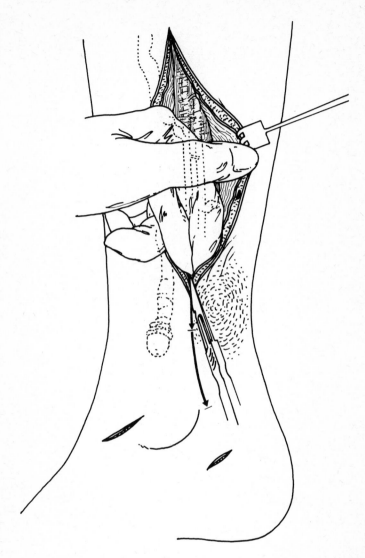

Fig. 68. By inserting two fingers under the deep fascia, it can be lifted off the underlying muscle, and then incised step by step between the fingers.

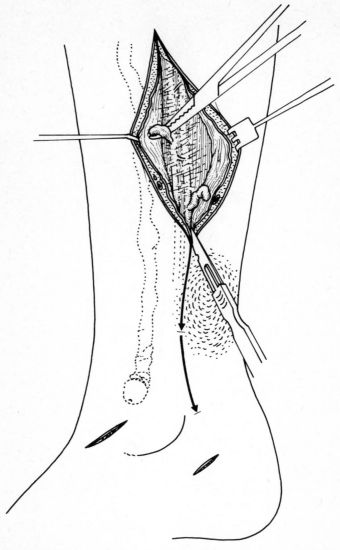

Fig. 69. *The perforating veins can be seen and picked up as they pass from the posterior tibials, penetrate the deep fascia from its deep aspect on their way to the great saphenous.*

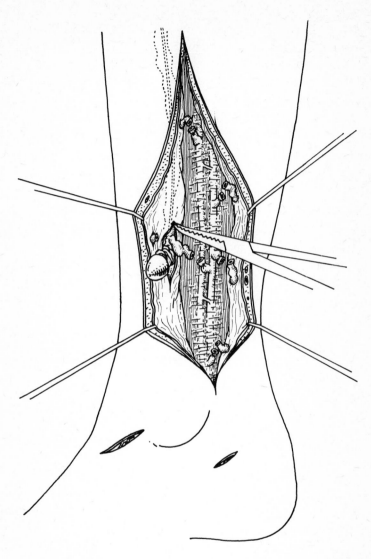

Fig. 70. A stuck stripper head may also be approached from the deep aspect of the deep fascia.

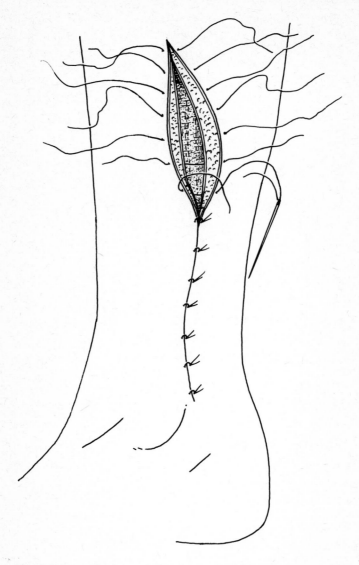

Fig. 71. The skin and fascia are closed as a single layer, with interrupted si sutures.

CHAPTER 17

The Treatment of Venous Ulcer

A venous ulcer will virtually always heal with effective and sufficiently prolonged elevation of the leg. Presumably this works by relieving the venules and arterio-venous capillaries of the extra distending effect of hydrostatic pressure. This would allow those that had become dilated, to contract down again and cease to be the preferred routes described. But the ulcer usually recurs again soon after ambulation has been resumed. Elevation of the leg means a horizontal position of the leg in relation to the heart. It is relatively ineffective if the patient's thorax is propped up with pillows, though there is no advantage in refusing the patient a pillow for his head.

Permanent elevation is obviously impracticable, but elevation for as much of the day as possible is very much better than none. Half elevation, as on a chair while sitting, is also better than nothing, but not so good as half as long fully recumbent. Every other measure aiming to reduce or combat excessive capillary pressure is employed. The most readily available method is compression (see Chapter 5).

The first step surgically is to relieve the venous cause of poor microcirculation, as described in the previous chapter. If this is able to be done effectively, healing of the ulcer is likely to follow; but the healing of a large area from the edges may take a long time. It can often be greatly hastened by skin grafting. Many surgeons have tried treating venous ulcers by laying a skin graft directly on to an ulcer base, even without preliminary attention to varicose veins, when present.

However, to expect an area of tissue to support grafted skin when it could not even maintain epithelium that had grown there naturally in the first place, seems to us illogical. It could have been done only on the basis of a notion that it had been the skin that had in some way been at fault, rather than the circulation of the subcutaneous tissue. So effective is elevation that such a graft may take and survive, but usually for little longer than the patient remains recumbent.

The next step after doing all one can for the venous condition is to provide the best possible bed for the graft. This is done by **wide excision**

of the ulcer. The excisions should be taken well into relatively healthy tissue, and down to, but **not including deep fascia**. This may mean excising to a depth of 2 or 3 cm in what is often a thick and sometimes oedematous leg. Fascia itself provides a moderately good bed for a skin graft, but better still—much, in our view—is that offered by healthy granulation tissue. Each granule of this represents a new capillary loop, and the excellent blood supply is demonstrated by the ease with which it can be made to bleed.

It has been no surprise, therefore, to find delayed grafting, a few days after the excision of the ulcer, to be so much the most successful method. There is no need to wait for granulations to grow flush with surrounding skin, for the crater left by early grafting fills out in due course anyway. Moreover, the longer the delay between excision and grafting, the greater the chance of infection becoming established. Indeed, it is better if the dressing on the site of excision can be left undisturbed until grafting.

Granulations are in the best state to receive a graft when they are deep pink or red and virtually free from exudate. The graft is a Thiersch, or split-skin graft, which has the highest take rate and is the only kind suitable for the area and the purpose. It is cut with a razor, is 1 to 1·5 mm thick, and takes off the tips of the dermal papillae, the layer from which regeneration takes place. Thus healing of the donor site begins all over, and is complete in 8 or 10 days, no matter how large the graft. The graft contains no elastic tissue and does not shrink. But it does curl or roll up. This is easily prevented if it is spread immediately, skin side down on to paraffin gauze, which is then applied to the bed. The depression is then packed with more paraffin gauze until this is proud, and then firmly bandaged. It is important that the graft be kept firmly pressed against the base.

In some category B ulcers in older subjects with varicose veins associated with the ulcer, the veins are occasionally considered suitable for injection. In this case nothing surgical is done to the ulcer until the whole response to sclerotherapy is quite complete—usually about six weeks. By then the ulcer is often healed, though one in three breaks down again within three years, and will then have to come to excision. In other category B ulcers in which varicose veins are dealt with surgically, the ulcer may be excised at the same time and grafted later as described above.

In an atypical category A case in which the skin is relatively healthy and the ulcer not too large, surgical excision of veins elsewhere in the leg may suffice and the ulcer may become healed with no more than a compressive bandage.

We believe *all* category A ulcers (younger subjects) to be postphlebitic, though only 70 per cent are reported to have clear evidence of it at radiography. The same treatment is used for these ulcers.

Mixed ulcers with an arteriosclerotic element

Improving the venous drainage might reasonably be expected to benefit the circulation and improve arterial blood supply. But no treatment of mixed ulcers has a high success rate. In the presence of arterial disease, wounds, particularly in the lower limb, will not heal, and excision of an ulcer cannot be considered. And the elevation that so improves the prospect of healing in pure venous ulcer, makes all the results of arterial disease worse. The best that can be tried is getting the ulcer as bacteriologically clean as possible with frequent bathing or irrigation with very weak solutions of sodium hyperchlorite, and powdering with an antibiotic. This is combined with supporting the leg in the position of partial elevation best tolerated by the patient. When optimum conditions appear to have been reached, pinch grafts are applied. These are taken from the arm; lest donor sites on a leg should not heal properly. Firm dressings are not tolerated and should be avoided. Ointments of any kind often do more harm than good.

CHAPTER 18

The Treatment of Lymphoedema, Erysipelas, Non-vascular Oedema, and Lipoedema

LYMPHOEDEMA

All lymphoedemas are treated alike, regardless of cause. Indeed, they have in the past all been assumed to have a similar cause, namely, a simple mechanical failure of lymph drainage. Most of the conservative measures routinely employed do usually slightly improve the swelling, though, as we hope to show, probably not for the reasons commonly supposed. In fact, in our view, nothing has yet been discovered which effectively controls the cause. The treatment of lymphoedema is therefore essentially palliative.

For lymphoedema with mild swelling conservative methods are used alone. For those with more severe or recalcitrant swelling, surgical methods are available. These fall into two groups: operations aimed to provide alternative drainage routes for lymph, and simple excisions of the 'target organ', the tissue in which the lymphoedema accumulates. Unfortunately all these drainage operations have been so unsuccessful that they have brought all surgery for lymphoedema into disrepute. This is a pity, for the results of excision of the oedematous subcutaneous tissue have been satisfactory and lasting (Fig. 72).

According to modern concepts of lymphoedema, operations designed to persuade a watery solution to leave the limb by an artificial route were doomed to fail; for they started from a false premise, namely that mechanical obstruction to the drainage of a watery solution was the fundamental trouble. However, there is no mechanical barrier to the excretion of water. For normally **all** water that is diffused outwards from capillary walls and is not used to form lymph, diffuses back again into the plasma. It is not retention of *water* that directly results from defective

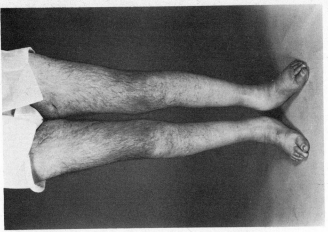
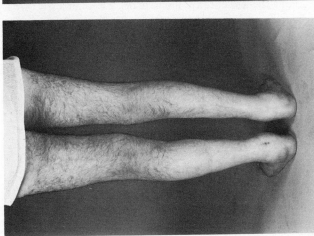
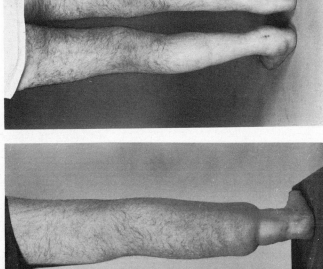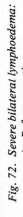

Fig. 72. *Severe bilateral lymphoedema:*
  A. *Before operation.*
  B. *Three years after operation.*
  C. *Excisions alone on the right; Thompson's combined operation on the left.*

lymph drainage, but retention of *protein*. Being at a lower concentration in interstitial fluid than in plasma, retained protein is bound to accumulate in the tissues until its concentration is equal to that in the plasma. Only then can directionally balanced diffusion of protein into the capillaries take place, and no further accumulation of protein in the tissues occur. Thus the water of lymphoedema may be said to be held in the tissues by the osmotic action of the protein, and obviously offering this water an additional pathway by which to leave the limb is irrelevant and useless. Any hope that the proteins might drain by the alternative route was in fact disappointed.

Many people still imagine that elevation encourages water to leave the leg rather as it is poured out of a jug. Such a naïve picture leads them to misunderstand none-the-less effective manœuvres. Elevation does help by dramatically reducing capillary blood pressure. Thus a proportion of the excess osmotic pressure of the retained protein is counterbalanced and some of the water is able to diffuse into the capillaries. The lymphoedema is slightly reduced. Compression works, as it does in venous oedema, by increasing the effective interstitial-fluid pressure; and diuretics work by concentrating the blood and increasing its osmotic pressure. All these measures are very much less effective in lymphoedema than in venous oedema.

The conservative management of lymphoedema

When the lymphoedema is first diagnosed the patient is, if possible, admitted to hospital to assess how much can be achieved by conservative methods. Fluid intake and output are measured. The volume of the limb is measured by water displacement, and recorded. The following regime is instituted in hospital.

1. The foot of the bed is raised at least 20 cm, and pillows put under the leg. The thorax must not be propped up, but there is no objection to a pillow for the patient's head.

2. Intermittent compression of the leg or legs by Flowtron leggings is applied for 12 hours out of 24.

3. Firm compression by crêpe bandage is applied at all other times. Less pressure is tolerated by the recumbent patient than by an ambulant one, but as much as the patient finds comfortable is used.

4. A diuretic, Lasix, 40 mg is given daily for three days.

5. If insufficient improvement is achieved it may be considerably increased by the following technique. Very powerful compression is applied to the leg by winding on a stout 1 cm wide rubber tube from the toes up. This acts like an arterial tourniquet, and unless done quickly and

removed, it can become agonizingly painful. Moreover, it is much too dangerous to use under anaesthesia. Skin rupture can occur, and ischaemic skin necrosis can result. But the method is remarkably effective and some patients tolerate it well (Van der Molen, 1962).

Long-term conservative management

If it is decided to continue conservative management, this has to be life long. It means reorganizing the patient's whole life, which in future must revolve around his disease. He must be seen every 12 months or so for reassessment of progress, and water-displacement measurement of limb volume, so that such modifications may be made in his regime as are indicated. The following may be tried in the first place.

1. As much of every day as possible is spent in complete recumbency. Time spent sitting with the limb on a chair is better than ordinary dependency; but half as long in complete recumbency is better.

2. Flowtron leggings are worn at night and for the odd hour whenever possible.

3. Well-fitting elastic stockings are worn whenever the patient is upright.

4. Massage helps some patients and is comforting.

5. Bathing is an excellent pastime, for the legs are compressed in proportion to their depth below the surface of the water. That is often in proportion to the hydrostatic pressure in blood vessels at all levels. Swimming should, therefore, be encouraged.

Long-term diuretics have side-effects and are not recommended.

Surgery for lymphoedema

We cannot recommend any of the so-called 'drainage operations' for lymphoedema, because we have not found one that worked. We also believe them all to be based on mistaken theory. Before appreciating this, one of us did indeed try several of these, particularly the combined drainage and excisional technique of Thompson (1971). In some cases of bilateral lymphoedema the combined operation was used on one side, and excision alone on the other. No superiority could be detected on the side having the addition of the drainage procedure (Fig. 72).

When excision of oedematous subcutaneous tissue was first practised by Sir Robert Charles in 1912, everything was removed including the skin, down to and also including the deep fascia. The bare muscles were then covered with free skin grafts. Complete loss of subcutaneous tissue frequently led to gangrene of the toes. Also the grafts provided an unsatisfactory, thin, pigmented, vulnerable and unsightly surface. The modern tendency is to preserve the skin and a thin layer of subcutaneous tissue, by making multi-stage excisions beneath skin flaps.

The technique of operation for lymphoedema

The preparation of the skin, towelling and instruments, are as for varicose-vein surgery (see Chapter 14), with the addition to the instruments of a Kidde's inflatable tourniquet and 8 Redivac drains. A Kidde's tourniquet is like a sphygmomanometer cuff and is inflated sufficiently to arrest arterial bleeding.

The excisions are done in 3 stages separated by 2 or 3 months, thus:

1. The medial half of the thigh and leg.
2. The lateral half of the thigh and leg.
3. The dorsum of the foot (Fig. 73).

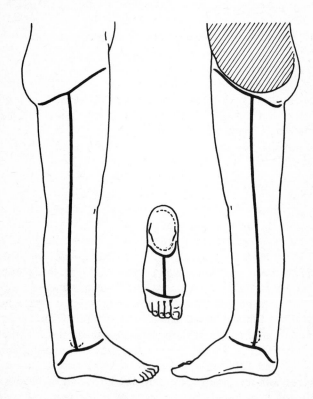

Fig. 73. The incisions for all three stages of the operation for lymphoedema.

At the upper end the incisions follow the groin crease and the sub-gluteal crease. In obese patients they run parallel with, but a centimetre or two below the actual creases. Towards its lateral end the groin incision turns horizontally at a level determined by the amount of involvement in this area, for this varies a good deal from patient to patient. In fact normal women often develop unsightly pads of fat over the great trochanters, which many plastic surgeons will remove for them as a cosmetic procedure. However, the swelling of lymphoedema tends to fade away towards the upper and outer limits. Indeed, particularly in older patients, stage 2 may even on occasion be omitted altogether.

Stage 1

The Kidde's tourniquet is applied as high as possible in the thigh, and inflated to a pressure of 200 or 300 mm Hg to occlude the arteries.

An incision about half a cm deep is made in the midline of the medial aspect of the thigh and leg, from just below the tourniquet to below the medial malleolus. At the lower end this is carried forward to the middle of the ankle anteriorly, and backwards to the middle of the Achilles tendon, as shown in Fig. 73. (Nothing further is done at the upper end yet.)

Flaps of skin *with 3 mm of subcutaneous fat* are raised to the midlines of the back and front of the leg (Fig. 74). There is an almost irresistible tendency to make the flaps thinner as one approaches their bases. It is so important that this be avoided, and so much better to err on the side of thickening the flaps, that a deliberate effort is made to thicken the flaps to 5 mm towards the bases.

The original incisions are now deepened down to and just through the deep fascia. The fascia can be lifted off the underlying muscle very much more easily than the fat can be dissected off the deep fascia; also the muscle provides a better bed, more richly supplied with blood, for the skin flaps, than fascia.

Two masses of oedematous fat corresponding with the skin flaps are now excised, using a temporary horizontal cut just below the tourniquet (Fig. 75). **All** veins, including the two saphenous veins, are ligated and divided as encountered, in stages 1 and 2. The saphenous and sural nerves accompanying the two saphenous veins are sacrificed, but the cutaneous branch of the peroneal is preserved if possible.

The Kidde's tourniquet is deflated (but not removed) and haemostasis is everywhere obtained with diathermy, or 0000 chromic catgut, but bearing in mind that **extensively** burned tissue does not make a good bed. The next step is trimming of redundant skin and suture of the skin of the lower leg to just above the knee. First the skin may be very roughly trimmed, erring, of course, on the side of moderate removal. Next one

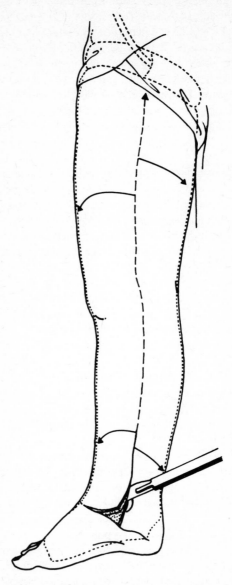

Fig. 74. Stage 1: two skin flaps are raised.

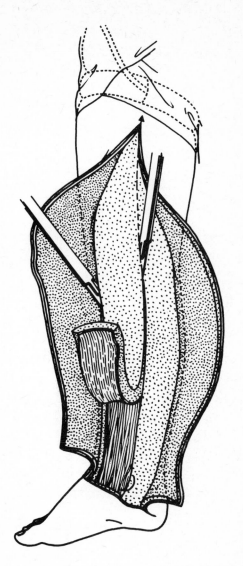

Fig. 75. Corresponding areas of deep fascia and oedematous fat are excised.

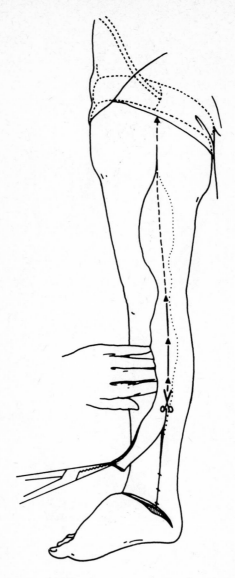

Fig. 76. The Kidde's tourniquet has been deflated. Final trimming of the lower
two-thirds of the skin, and suture is completed.

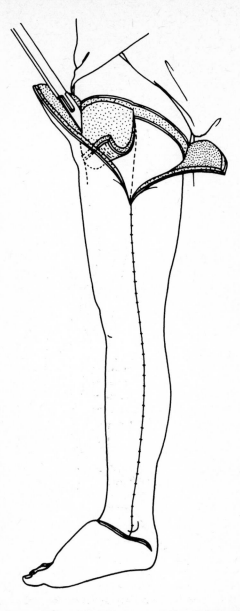

Fig. 77. The Kidde's tourniquet has been removed and the patient retowelled. The top incisions have been made and the top-most part of the fat excisions are being completed.

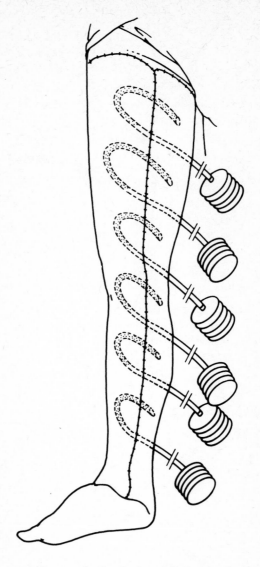

Fig. 78. Showing the distribution of the Redivac drains.

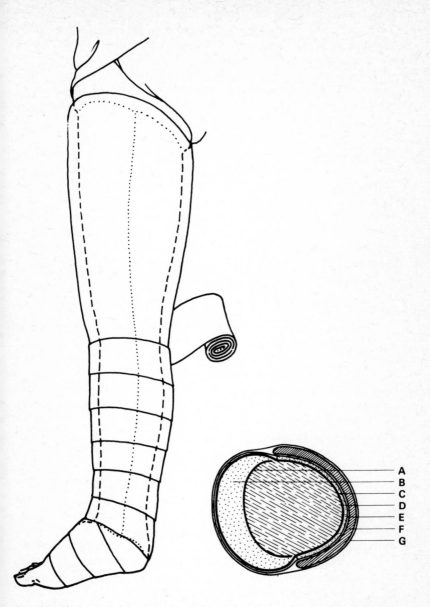

Fig. 79. The wounds have been dressed and the plaster-of-paris slabs are being bandaged in position. A. Deep facia. B. Oedematous subcutaneous tissue. C. Skin. D. Gauze and cotton wool. E. Crêpe bandage. F. Plaster-of-paris. G. Crêpe bandage.

flap overlaps the other, and the underneath one is sewn to the other with interrupted 000 silk mattress sutures tied only tight enough to give what is felt to be normal skin tension. Final, accurate trimming will now be found much easier (Fig. 76).

The final trim and skin sutures are done in stages, each about 10 cm long and each completed before the next is started. The suture is done both with interrupted 000 silk and with continuous 0000 monofil nylon. At this point the tourniquet is completely removed. After this the skin is reprepared and the patient retowelled as necessary. The top ends of the skin incisions are now completed, and the removal of the rest of the fat (Fig. 77). It will be found that there is less thickness to remove here as the thickening fades away at the upper end and towards the outer side. Finally the trimming of the skin and suturing are also completed. It is nearly always found that the flaps need to be pulled upwards somewhat, as well as overlapped, and that a triangle of skin has to be excised at the top edge of each flap. All the way along the skin suture, as it proceeds, Redivac drains will have been distributed, making a total of 6 or 8, each draining both sides as shown (Fig. 78).

Dressing (Fig. 79)

The dressing of this very large operation site is an important part of the operation, and should always be done by the operating surgeon himself. For a good result it is essential that even pressure should be achieved all over the area. First the suture lines are covered with pieces of tulle gras and gauze. Next an even layer of cotton-wool is applied and held in position with a sterile crêpe bandage. Finally, plaster-of-paris slabs, each 8 layers thick, are spread over the whole and bandaged in place with crêpe bandage.

Aftercare

While still in, the drains should be occasionally checked to make sure that they are working properly and maintaining their vacuums. The colour of the toes is inspected to make sure that no bandage is too tight.

Unless they are still draining freely, the drains are removed on the third day and ambulation starts.

Some of the interrupted sutures are removed on the 10th day and the plaster-of-paris slabs discarded. The rest and the continuous suture are left as long as possible, up to, say, another week.

Stage 2

The thickening is much less marked on the outer side, particularly towards the upper end of the thigh. In older people the lateral stage may even be omitted altogether, and the dorsum of the foot dealt with second.

For stage 2 the Kidde's tourniquet is applied as for stage 1. In the first place the incision is carried from a short way below the tourniquet to below the lateral malleolus, in the midline of the lateral aspect of the thigh and lower leg. At the lower end it is continued forward to the midline anteriorly, and back to the middle of the Achilles tendon. As previously, skin flaps 4 mm thick (i.e. with 3 mm of fat) are raised to the midlines anteriorly and posteriorly.

The incisions are now deepened just through the deep fascia, step-by-step as before, and the fascia and oedematous fat excised over an area corresponding to the skin flaps. The Kidde's tourniquet is removed and haemostasis secured. The skin has now been uncovered for the completion of the upper end. How high the excision is to be carried varies somewhat with the requirements of each patient. Usually the skin incision reaches to about the tip of the great trochanter. The groin crease is followed from the end of the scar left from stage 1 and turns horizontally where decided. The posterior cut meets the previous scar in the subgluteal crease. The excisions of fat, trimming of the skin, drainage and suture, are completed and aftercare carried out as described for stage 1.

Stage 3 (Fig. 80)

Though the smallest area, this is the most time consuming.

The Kidde's tourniquet is applied in the thigh. The two scars between the tips of the two malleoli are excised. An incision at right angles to this is carried nearly to the base of the toes, in the midline of the foot. Incisions extend from the end of this, medially and laterally to the margins of the foot. The oedematous subcutaneous fat is excised as previously, but this time the whole of the superficial venous arch must be preserved. If it is not so, the toes are apt to become oedematous. Skin repair is completed as previously, with two Redivac drains as shown (Fig. 80D).

THE TREATMENT OF ERYSIPELAS

The patient is confined to bed so long as there is fever or he still feels sick. Penicillin is given in doses usually described as 'massive'. One million units are given intramuscularly daily for 2 or 3 days, followed by 3 or 4 days of oral dosage at more usual levels.

Erysipelas is contagious and the local lesion should be kept covered. An ointment containing a local anaesthetic and an antibiotic, such as Nebactin and Gramacidin is useful.

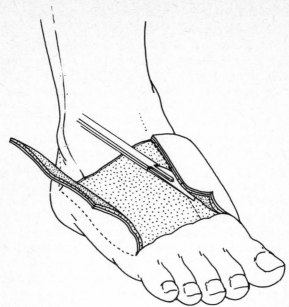

Fig. 80. Stage 3. A. The second skin flap on the dorsum of the foot is being turned back.

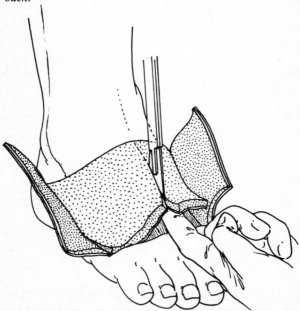

B. The oedematous fat is being lifted and dissected off.

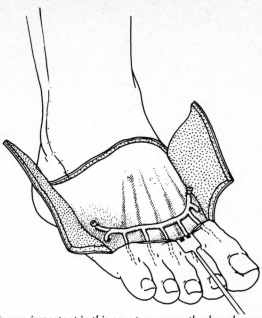

C. It is very important in this case to preserve the dorsal venous arch.

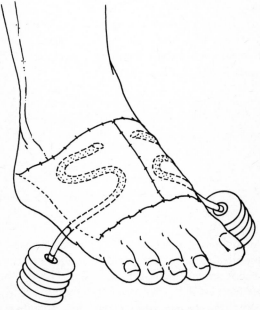

D. The skin incision has been closed and Redivac drains left in.

Prophylactic treatment

Recurrent attacks of erysipelas are a sufficiently common complication of lymphoedema to justify extended prophylactic measures. These may take the form of long-acting sulphonamides (so that only one dose per day is required). One of us has had success with a slightly modified version of the method of Konopik, a contemporary Czech dermatologist. The following mixture is infiltrated subcutaneously 4 or 5 times, in the area affected.

Hyaluronidase, 3,000 U.
Lignocaine 0·5 per cent with adrenalin, 10 ml.
Heparin, 5,000 U.
Normal saline for I.V. use, 50 ml.

The injections are repeated every 2 or 3 days, and throughout the treatment a daily dose of iron and vitamin C are given. The treatment is always started during remission.

NON-VASCULAR OEDEMA

When a patient is referred with a diagnosis of non-vascular oedema the consultant is not absolved of the responsibility for making sure that no other cause for oedema, such as renal or cardiac disease, has been overlooked. When the diagnosis of non-vascular oedema is beyond doubt, the most important aspect of management lies in doing everything possible to increase the patient's physical activity of all kinds. The best sport is swimming, because bathing involves an element of compression of the legs. Indeed, the compression is in proportion to the depth below the surface. When the patient stands collar-bone deep, compression is in proportion to the hydrostatic pressure in the blood vessels, at all levels. If activity has been limited by pain, this must be properly controlled with such drugs as aspirin or phenyl butazolidine. If the patient has a condition such as painful flat feet, hammer toes, or bunions, or pain in the back, the assistance of an orthopaedic or rheumatological colleague is likely to be called for.

In addition to more general increase in physical activity, more specific exercises are often required. These should include exercises designed to improve venous circulation; such as rising on the toes and deep breathing. If the swelling is not completely controlled by these simple measures, or if the patient presses for some additional 'magic', the Flowtron leggings may be applied for a couple of hours a day (or night) with spectacular results. Compression, prolonged elevation, and diuretics are seldom needed and may be held in reserve.

For the cases where the swelling is associated with menstruation, particularly when dysmenorrhoea is also present, gynaecological investigation may be indicated. Psychoneurosis and depression are also watched for so that suitable management may be arranged.

Prophylactic treatment for Traveller's Ankle

We hold this condition to be the result of restricted activity of the calf pump. One of us has, therefore, suggested that passengers in coaches or aeroplanes should make a point of flexing and extending the toes and ankles two or three times every half hour. Some results are reported in the Appendix, no. 7.

LIPOEDEMA OR LIPIDOSIS

Nothing can be done in the early stages of diffuse swelling of the legs, beyond attention to any superadded non-vascular oedema. At a much later stage the fat tends to become regionalized. It may then be excised in large masses. So excised, the fat does not tend to reappear, and the patient is often inordinately grateful for what she considers some return towards normality.

Wide excisions have been opposed on the grounds that they would involve destruction of many normal lymphatic trunks and might cause lymphoedema. No such sequel has occurred in our hands.

Treatment of Leg Swelling in Pregnancy

1. Deep venous thrombosis

Any swelling of sudden onset during pregnancy or the puerperium, particularly if preceded by pain and associated with tenderness in a muscle, should be assumed to be due to spontaneous deep venous thrombosis and requires immediate confirmation and treatment. The management is described in Chapter 16. Radio-active isotopes are contra-indicated in pregnancy, but phlebography is not. Heparin may be used with care, having first made sure that protamine sulphate is on hand. The cumarins are strictly avoided.

2. Varicose veins and spider veins

With modern anaethesia, surgery is not contra-indicated in pregnancy and can achieve good results (Haeger, 1968); nor must treatment by injection of sclerosants be avoided (Sigg, 1963). However, there are two good reasons for doing no more than what is immediately necessary: one is the expectation of some spontaneous improvement after childbirth; the other that, if the mother has the misfortune to have a 'spastic' or a 'mongol', the treatment is sure to be blamed. The doctor may ease his own conscience with the thought that he was certainly not to blame, but the parents may never forgive themselves for having agreed to the treatment. Above all, spider veins are left alone till later.

3. Lymphoedema

There is never any urgency about the treatment of lymphoedema which, at the worst, is a very chronic and slowly progressing disease. If a pre-existing lymphoedema seems to be getting worse, probably because of super-added non-vascular oedema, an elastic stocking is applied and daily rests in recumbency advised.

4. Non-vascular oedema

To the extent that this is due to hormonally-induced water retention, nothing can be done, except to reassure the patient that it will disappear after birth of the child. However, some of the ankle oedema may be due to inadequate exercise of the accessory venous pumps. Patients who get leg swelling during pregnancy should therefore make a practice of frequently lifting themselves on the toes, and taking 2 or 3 deep breaths.

Appendices

1

NOTES ON MORTALITY FROM PULMONARY EMBOLISM

When deep venous thrombosis has a fatal outcome, the usual cause of death is lodging of a blood clot in a main pulmonary artery, sometimes immediately killing the patient, sometimes leading to death via pneumonia. The figures for deaths certified as having been due to pulmonary embolism given in the Registrar General's Statistical Review for England and Wales therefore serve as an index of what is happening in deep venous thrombosis in Britain. According to this review, 2,687 people were certified as having died from pulmonary embolism during 1971, which represents a rate of 55 per million of living population. This rate has been rising relatively steadily year by year in the eleven years for which we have figures (Table 1). Such a regular increase calls for an equally regularly operating cause.

The first explanation that suggests itself is that the figures reflect increasing awareness of the condition and progressive improvement in diagnostic techniques, until we remember that the diagnosis of pulmonary embolism is perhaps most often made at necropsy and is not likely to have been greatly affected by such factors. Perhaps the fatality figures do no more than reflect the increasing proportion of patients that are being subjected to surgical operations, the increasing age at which the patients are undergoing operation, and the increasing severity and length of procedures being undertaken. Another, to us less convincing notion is that the trend is related to increasing use of the relaxants.

Whatever the cause of the trend, the figures certainly show no evidence suggesting the introduction of a much more effective method of treatment or of prophylaxis, such as might be hoped for should intermittent compression win wide adoption as a routine prophylactic method (see Appendix, no. 9).

TABLE 1

Number of deaths certified as due to
pulmonary embolism

England and Wales

	Number	Rate per million population
1961	1645	36
1962	1711	37
1963	1906	41
1964	1976	42
1965	2006	42
1966	2195	46
1967	2408	50
1968	2410	50
1969	2447	50
1970	2659	54
1971	2687	55

Registrar General's Statistical Review, England and Wales, 1971, Part I. London: H.M.S.O., 1973.

2

BASIC COMPRESSION

As Barron (1960) pointed out, the volume of the blood substantially exceeds what would be the total capacity of the cardiovascular system if all the vessels were in an unstretched state. In other words, its elastic vessels are in a constant state of considerable distension against their elastic walls. Or, as Starling wrote in 1909, paraphrasing what he had previously referred to as 'the classical paper of Weber' (Bayliss and Starling, 1894), 'If the circulation were brought to a standstill, the pressure in all parts of the system would be the same. This is called the mean systemic pressure.'

Starling went on: 'If the circulation be re-established by means of the heart-pump . . . on the venous side the pressure will sink below the mean systemic pressure; on the arterial side the pressure will be raised above the mean pressure.' That is, arterial pressure is mean systemic pressure plus an effect of cardiac action, and venous pressure is mean systemic pressure *minus* the effect of escape of venous blood into the diastolic heart. Though he did not say so, this would have implied that the raised venous pressure of heart failure represented a return towards mean systemic pressure, rather than being due to the continued arrival of venous blood at a rate faster than it was being removed by the failing heart (a naïve notion still much current long after Starling's day). It could only have arisen from imagining the cardiovascular system as including an *open* reservoir at the venous end. (This is the way it was then customarily illustrated—and still sometimes is.) In a closed system the volume of venous return can differ from that of cardiac output by an amount equal to any change occurring in total vascular capacity, and cardiac output can differ from the volume entering the heart to the extent that the volume of blood remaining in the heart after systole, changes.

By using the word 'mean' in mean systemic pressure, Starling gave the impression that he felt it should lie midway between arterial and venous pressure. But what he had described would not, in fact, do so. This was illustrated by one of us when writing about venous pressure (Johnson, 1964). This is because if the circulation were brought to rest, venous pressure would rise and arterial pressure would fall. Some blood would be transferred from arteries to veins. However, this would require less dilatation of veins *proportionally* than it would involve constriction of arteries. As shown in the experiment described, arterial pressure would fall more than venous pressure would rise. The level at which arterial and venous pressure finally became equalized would therefore be closer to what venous than to what arterial pressure had been.

In the paper (Johnson, 1964), an entity called 'basic compression' was described. This was defined as 'the pressure at which arterial and venous pressure would become equalized soon after the circulation had been brought to rest if it had been possible to "freeze" the calibres of every vessel in the body immediately before such arrest'. The definition would have better fitted Starling's phrase; for it *would* have stood midway between arterial and venous pressure. That it would do so was also illustrated by the experiment. For when the circuit of a pump-and-tube model was made of rigid tubing, stopping the pump caused the resulting fall in output pressure and rise in inlet pressure to be exactly equal in extent. 'Freezing' the calibre of the vessels is the same as converting them notionally to a rigid system. We hold that basic compression is a more realistic index of the overall effect of vascular compression than Starling's 'mean systemic pressure'. Moreover, we believe Starling himself would have preferred it when the defect in his own definition had been demonstrated to him by the experiment described.

Basic pressure and compression and their origins

Compression may be defined as the fluid pressure in the contents of a distended elastic tube, due to tension in its wall. When the calibre of a tube is not in actual process of changing, the compression by its walls and the fluid pressure in its contents must, of course, be the same. 'Basic compression' is therefore *numerically* equal to basic pressure, but they are not the same thing. Basic pressure is the pressure which keeps the vessels distended. Basic compression is derived partly from tension in inert elastic fibres, and partly from active muscle tone.

Basic pressure arises from the operation of the net osmotic pressure of plasma proteins drawing fluids from the interstitial compartment into the capillaries. At first glance it might be guessed that, since this is its origin, basic pressure must be equal to net osmotic pressure, and so it would have been if the blood had been stationary, with pressure everywhere the same. However, as was shown in Appendix no. 5, the net osmotic pressure of plasma protein is about 18 mm Hg, while the basic pressure and compression, as here defined, are nearer 60 mm Hg. But when the blood is circulating, it is only pressure in the capillaries with which net osmotic pressure would be in balance. If it had been the great veins that had been semi-permeable, for instance, instead of the capillaries, it would have been here that blood pressure and osmotic pressure would have been equal, and basic pressure, venous pressure and arterial pressure would all have been much higher than they are.

3

ELECTRICAL ANALOGUES VERSUS PUMP-AND-TUBE MODELS IN THE STUDY OF CARDIOVASCULAR MECHANICS

Ten years ago one of us wrote a paper on venous pressure (Johnson, 1964) which began with the words: 'In this paper I have begun by describing some experiments with simple mechanical models. This is not because I imagine that they prove anything physiological, nor because it is possible to deduce from them reactions to be expected from an exceedingly complicated multiple-feed-back machine such as the cardio-vascular system. They *illustrate* certain fundamental principles which govern the behaviour of a passively-filling pump connected in a ring circuit with a system of elastic tubes—principles which may not be assumed to have no influence on physiological events.' Nevertheless, an editorial in a leading medical journal described the paper as 'an attempt to prove with models', and evidently the writer considered that these words justified him in discarding the conclusions drawn.

At that time it was and for all we know still is, fashionable to sneer at mechanical models and to prefer what were called 'electrical analogues'. Perhaps the flow of liquids in tubes does bear a very superficial resemblance to the flow of an electrical current in a simple circuit; and the laws which relate to flow in systems in parallel and in series are roughly similar for liquids and electricity, provided one does not insist too much on precise definition of terms. However, there the similarity ends; and a physicist who learned of this curious preference might be forgiven for concluding that those who used electrical analogues could not have got further than Ohm's Law in electricity, or have heard about Laplace, Poiseuille or Bernouil in fluid mechanics.

A pressure head could be said roughly to correspond with voltage; but there is nothing in electricity to correspond with hydrostatic pressure or with syphonage, both of such importance in physiology. The laws which govern the relationship between the calibre of a tube and its resistance to flow of a liquid do not remotely resemble those which relate the thickness of a wire to its resistance to an electric current. All moving liquids have rates of volume flow which could be said to correspond with amperage; but they also vary in their velocities of flow, which electric currents in simple circuits do not. There is nothing whatever in electricity to correspond with viscosity, or osmotic pressure, or side pressure and end

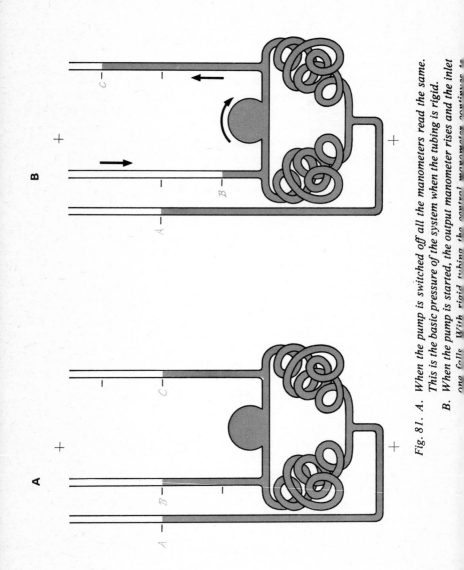

Fig. 81. A. When the pump is switched off all the manometers read the same.
This is the basic pressure of the system when the tubing is rigid.
B. When the pump is started, the output manometer rises and the inlet
one falls. With rigid tubing the central manometer continues to

pressure, or the Bernouil effect; neither can the sigma effect nor axial accumulation of cells, or laminar flow, be imitated electrically; nor is there anything in fluid mechanics to resemble magnetism or electrical inductance.

No doubt by exercise of great ingenuity electricians will manage to make electrical analogues behave in ways faintly representing some of the features of liquid behaviour mentioned; but what would be the point? Why this extraordinary reluctance to accept that far the best way to begin to understand the events that can be observed in the cardio-vascular system is by mastering the behaviour of Newtonian liquids in simple tube-and-pump models.

One of us once heard a professor of cardiology say: 'I have been sitting all night with a wet towel round my head trying to understand why giving so-and-so, which is known to be a vasodilator, has the effect of raising venous pressure.' It happened that the effect which he described was exactly that which would have been expected on the basis of observation of the simplest of tube-and-pump models.

4

COMPARISON OF HUMAN LEG WITH HIND LEG OF A DOG

So much physiological and medical research is being carried out on dogs that it is important to appreciate that there are considerable differences, and that unless these are kept constantly in mind one is apt to arrive at conclusions which do not necessarily operate in man.

The most obvious differences between a human leg and the hind leg of a dog arise from their difference of posture. In the dog the femur is held much flexed at the hip joint, with the knee close to the lower ribs. The range of movement at the knee is small and it remains flexed to about 90°. The homologue of the human heel is held well off the ground, and the dog walks, as it were, on its toes. The metatarsals, which form part of the foot in man, are represented by what feels like a single bone but is really a bundle of four. (The dew-claw represents the 5th metatarsal.) Ordinarily the capillary pressure to be coped with in the feet on standing is not nearly so high as that in man. Nevertheless, the dog seems perfectly capable of adjusting to the requirements of upright stance, yet it has nothing resembling the venous calf pump of man. Indeed, not only are there no intra-muscular sinusoidal veins, but also there is no muscle remotely resembling the calf of man, for this has something like five times the bulk of the corresponding muscles in the dog.

Fat

Only some animals have a layer of fat between the skin and the deep fascia, and the dog is not one of them. Only in man does this layer vary so much in thickness from individual to individual, and only in man is the thickness of the layer altered by so many endocrine influences and even, it would seem, psychological ones.

Arteries

In the dog a prominent saphenous artery arises from the femoral artery in the adductor canal and follows the course of the popliteal artery in man. It then passes between the tibia and fibula, like the anterior tibial in man.

Veins

The veins of the leg in primates have changed a lot from those in quadrupeds. Dogs do not have the division into superficial and deep systems of the larger veins that is such a striking feature in the human leg, and no muscular veins similar to sinusoids in man are present. In dogs the short saphenous becoming the popliteal, is the main drainage channel of the leg, and the long saphenous is not a recognizable vein. In fact, few results of experimental work on the leg veins of a dog can be applied to man.

Lymphatics

The lymphatic systems of man and dog are much more alike, perhaps because there are no hydrostatic, gravitational effects on lymph. Man's upright stance would not, therefore, require the lymphatic system to undergo modification as it would the venous system. For instance, lymph pressure is higher at the groin than in the foot or paw of both dogs and man. Findings in experimental work on the lymphatic system in the dog may reasonably be expected to be the same as they would in man.

5

CALCULATION OF THE OSMOTIC PRESSURE OF THE INTERSTITIAL MATERIAL

So long as the partial pressures in fluids are the same on the two sides of a permeable membrane (hydraulic and osmotic together), diffusion through the membrane will be directionally balanced (but see reservation near the end of Chapter 5: in 'Formation and disposal at heart level'). Moreover, if the pressures are not equal diffusion in one direction will exceed that in the other. There is net outward or net inward diffusion (known as extravasation or absorption) through the walls of the capillaries, for instance, if the partial pressure of any particular fluid is different in the interstitial fluid from what it is in the blood plasma.

At the arterial ends of capillaries, and probably throughout capillaries with open sphincters at some levels, the hydraulic pressure greatly exceeds the osmotic pressure of the plasma proteins, and there must always be net outward diffusion of water and crystalloids there. This would cause progressive increase in osmotic attraction for interstitial fluid. At the same time, as the blood follows the pressure gradient along the capillary there would also be a progressive decline in hydraulic pressure. Net outward diffusion would similarly decline, halt, and give way to net inward diffusion. After this point reabsorption would exactly keep pace with continued change in osmotic and hydraulic pressures. There is no reason why the pressures should ever get out of equilibrium again (as they always seem to be asserted to do in physiology textbooks). Accordingly, at any point after the point of first equilibrium an equation may be written, thus:

Blood pressure − Interstitial-fluid pressure = Osmotic pressure of plasma proteins − Osmotic pressure of interstitial material

At the point where reabsorption comes to an end, the protein content of the blood must on the average be the same as it is in a main vein of the area. It is now believed that some reabsorption occurs even in venules, but the protein concentration cannot have changed much after leaving the venous ends of the capillaries. Accordingly the osmotic pressure of the plasma here will be taken as equal to that of arm-vein blood—about 25 mm Hg. Reasons have already been given for accepting the figure of Guyton et al. (1971) as the most dependable for interstitial-fluid pressure: that is 6 mm Hg below atmospheric pressure, or 754 mm Hg. The blood pressure at the venous ends of the capillaries has been many times measured directly, with results which have naturally varied. But the most popular average figure in textbooks of physiology seems to be 12 mm Hg relative to atmospheric pressure, of course, and is therefore equal to 772 mm Hg.

Using these figures brings the osmotic pressure of the interstitial material to 7 mm Hg, and the net osmotic pressure of the plasma proteins to 18 mm Hg. Referring to a figure calculated by Wiederhielm et al. (1970) for the osmotic pressure of the gel matrix, Guyton et al. (1971) happened to arrive at exactly the same figure.

6

SPECULATION CONCERNING THE TREATMENT OF THE POSTPHLEBITIC SYNDROME

Perhaps one day a valved, elastic tube will become available which can be implanted in the tissues to replace a blocked segment of deep vein, and itself remain unblocked. Meanwhile we hold that to put in a graft of superficial vein is useless unless some method is devised of preserving its nerve supply and muscular activity; for in some way the pumping activity of the normal deep venous system has to be restored or imitated.

We would suggest an alternative approach. This is that loss of main deep veins be accepted and that all blood be encouraged to go, instead, via the superficial veins, for if the patient survives the initial block, the blood can be depended on to find a new route for itself. However, for this to remain adequate without the usual secondary effects, it is necessary that the new routes should be provided with the external support and the intermittent compression hitherto peculiar to the deep veins.

Standing in water chest deep provides support to all submerged veins proportional to their depth beneath the surface of the water, that is to the hydrostatic pressure within them. Exactly the same effect could be achieved by applying a 'bandage' consisting of a long narrow cellophane bag, held in place with an inelastic bandage, and filled with water. The pressure of bandage compression can be adjusted by the simple device of attaching a tube to the top of the 'bag', taking it up to any level required, and filling it with water. The existing valves of the superficial veins are made use of, and the addition of a supply of intermittent pressure to the tube would establish a pumping mechanism, similar to the calf pump.

In order to prevent the very substantial pressure that would be applied at the lower end, from bursting the bag bandage, it would need to be inserted into a length of sock, like orthopaedic gauze. This in turn, would need to be supported by a stout, inelastic or very strongly elastic bandage. To make it easy to apply and less apt to slip, the 'bag' would need to be moulded on a bias, and wound on a slightly conical former, the 'sock' being attached to the upper, longer edge of the outside bandage. The bag bandage and its tube extension would be filled with water after application.

The intermittent pressure could be supplied by the same pump as already developed for the Flowtron legging, and it would not be difficult to construct a battery-driven model to make it portable.

7

TRAVELLER'S ANKLE: THE RESULTS OF THE SUGGESTED METHOD OF PROPHYLAXIS

One of us recently wrote to medical journals describing this condition, suggesting why it occurred and proposing a simple method of prophylaxis (all appearing in Chapter 18: Non-vascular Oedema). Doctors who decided to try the method suggested were asked to report their results. Many did write, nearly all recording success. Only two elderly sufferers noticed little improvement.

Another doctor reported that he had never suffered from Traveller's Ankle until he had acquired a car with an automatic gear change. Since then he had noticed swelling of the left ankle (only) after long car journeys. He attributed it to the left ankle no longer having anything to do. As others have pointed out, not every driver has this result, for many exercise the left leg more regularly after it has been freed of its clutch-operating duties.

Another doctor had been M.O. to a coach tour of Europe. On the outward journey five of his eighteen passengers had complained of painful swelling of the ankles. In Basle the doctor's attention had been drawn to one of the letters, and he had passed on its suggestion to his passengers. On the return journey none of the passengers had ankle swelling.

8

SPECULATION CONCERNING PERMEABILITY AND HOW THIS MIGHT BE DECREASED BY DEPENDENCY

One of us having advanced the suggestion that capillaries become less permeable in dependency, we have been asked 'How on earth could capillaries become *less* permeable when stretched?' This is not our 'field', and we would do no more than hazard a fanciful guess as to the direction in which the answer might lie. Stretching of capillaries would tend to increase their circumferential size, while leaving their lengths unaffected. Notionally round pores in their walls would, therefore, tend to become oval, with unchanged short axes and lengthened circumferential axes. With moving blood within, the capillaries might be judged to have static electrical charges on the outside. Around stomata that were oval in shape these charges would not remain evenly distributed. An asymmetrical molecule approaching a round stoma head on might be expected to pass through, while approaching an oval stoma surrounded by unevenly distributed charges, such a molecule might become reorientated across the stoma, and fail to pass.

9

FLOWTRON LEGGINGS

These consist of a pair of plastic leggings closed right down the front with buttons or zip fasteners. They extend from just below the knee to the base of the toes. Inside the strong outside skin is an inflatable lining of thinner plastic which, on inflation, compresses a leg enclosed within the legging. Attached to the legging is a small electrically-driven pump which inflates the linings alternately at a cycle of two to four minutes (1–2 min. inflated; 1–2 min. deflated), so that one is inflated while the other is collapsed. The pressure applied is adjustable, and can be varied from 20 to 65 mm Hg. The pump and motor weigh approximately 1·4 kg. They are driven from a mains supply and are double insulated, fully complying with Ministry safety requirements. A battery model is under development.

The object of intermittent compression of the legs

The effect of compression is to tend to squeeze blood in both directions out of all vessels in the region compressed. At the pressure applied, this will have little direct effect on larger arteries. Veins over about 2 mm in diameter are prevented from emptying retrogradely by their valves. Larger leg veins are therefore emptied proximally. Smaller veins empty easiest towards the ends where pressure is lowest; therefore even from valveless veins only a little retrograde emptying occurs. During the phase of relaxation of compression, larger veins cannot refill retrogradely, again because of their valves. Refilling is therefore entirely from the periphery. Smaller veins fill most easily from the ends where the pressure is highest; only a little retrograde refilling therefore occurs. Thus a venous pumping action results.

This pumping action is commonly imagined to exert its anti-thrombotic effect by increasing total blood flow through the limb and so combating venous stasis. However, this is not in accordance with what has since been shown to happen. We have repeatedly (Pflug, 1965a and b) drawn attention to the fact that it is in intramuscular veins that deep venous thrombosis nearly always starts. We have several times confirmed that when deep venous thrombosis occurs in a paraplegic or in an 'old polio', it is in the normal limb and not in the wasted, fibrotic one, with lost muscle sinusoids, that clotting is found to have begun. We have pointed out that, owing to the availability of alternative, easier routes for venous blood, little would be expected to go via intramuscular veins when circulation was low and no exercise of relevant muscles was taking place. Moreover, the muscle sinusoids are very wide as well as numerous. Accordingly, what little volume flow there was through them would cause minimal **velocity** of flow.

Accordingly, the original idea, by intermittent compression of the legs, was to **maintain circulation through the muscle sinusoids.** This was brought out in the publications mentioned above, but not in the first one reporting results (Hills, Pflug, Jeyasingh, Boardman, and Calnan, 1972). On other veins than muscle sinusoids, this pumping action would assist blood flow *while there was any*, but also altogether arrest flow during the phase of compression. Overall blood flow through the lower leg might well be diminished. The leggings could not, therefore, be expected to benefit a venous ulcer. However, in fact they do, though the reason is not yet clear. Moreover, so far only one length of cycle of inflation/deflation and one level of compression have been tried. It is surprising that so much success was achieved with these, and plainly much more experimental work remains to be done.

Another effect of intermittent compression is greatly to increase the flow of lymph. For a reason which we have not identified, the protein content of lymph from a limb under intermittent compression is **increased**. The Flowtron legging must therefore greatly increase excretion of protein from the tissue spaces. It would therefore have been expected greatly to benefit lymphatic oedema. The fact that it does so only to a limited extent suggests that the leggings must also increase extravasation of protein from the capillaries.

Results of prophylactic use

Bilateral pre-operative and post-operative intermittent compression is now carried out routinely on all patients undergoing operation from general surgical wards at Hammersmith Hospital (Royal Postgraduate Medical School). A survey of the results in 151 patients, made in conjunction with Barnet General Hospital, was completed and published in 1972 (Hills, Pflug, Jeyasingh, Boardman, and Calnan, 1972). It appeared that, except in malignant disease, the method could be depended on to bring about a very substantial reduction in the incidence of post-operative deep venous thrombosis, without side-effects. In the trial the reduction had been by about 90 per cent.

Effects on blood flow

More recent investigation has shown that intermittent compression, as applied in the test, greatly reduced total blood flow in the limb, and that this was accompanied by a well-marked rise in fibrinolytic activity. It was recalled that this has long been known to be an effect of exercise, and that the active material seems to be produced by vein walls. It was suggested that the second effect was caused by the first, and that this might be how the leggings worked (Allenby, Pflug, Boardman, and Calnan, 1973).

10

SAMPLE PAMPHLET FOR ISSUE TO ALL IN-PATIENTS IN HOSPITAL

Deep venous thrombosis is a painful condition of the leg which not uncommonly affects those lying still in hospital.

This can largely be prevented by moving the legs every now and again throughout the day.

When you are asleep you move enough without knowing it.

The condition is most apt to occur after big operations or difficult childbirths, and in the not so young.

Except during rest periods and at night, a bell will sound once (like a clock striking one) every half-hour.

When you hear it you should at least waggle your toes and ankles two or three times, and take two or three deep breaths. To move your other joints as well is also a good thing, but less essential.

If you are out of bed, you should walk round the ward while taking your deep breaths.

Please remind your neighbours to make their movements, particularly if they are elderly.

11

THE THEORETICAL BACKGROUND FOR MANAGEMENT OF VARICOSE VEINS

J. Pflug and H. Daintree Johnson

Paper read by invitation at the 1st American–European Symposium on Venous Diseases, Montreux, March 1974

Everyone undertaking the treatment of any disorder of veins will do so on the basis of the notion of its pathogenesis which he finds most convincing. Most of those current at the moment seem to be variants of the venostatic hypothesis: that is they regard **reduction of volume flow through main veins** as of paramount importance. Breakdown of valves, blockage of main deep veins and incompetence in perforating veins are taken to be pre-eminent features. We believe much that is now done and has been discussed today to have a good empirical basis. However, we find so much of the theory on which it is based to be inconsistent with observable fact as well as with elementary laws of fluid mechanics.

We should like to make a number of points where we shall offer alternative and we hope more convincing explanations. The first is an **anatomical** one. According to current teaching, the veins of the leg are divided into two distinct systems by deep fascia. Yet we all know that after stripping out both saphenous veins and tying all visible perforating veins, the superficial system continues to drain perfectly satisfactorily. Plainly, the most important channel connecting the superficial system to the deep must therefore be the vast network of the small to microscopic veins. Moreover, if amputated limbs are injected with Microfil—a material specially developed to fill capillaries—the superficial veins can be filled from the deep ones and the microscopic veins about and beneath the deep fascia are found to be in continuity right through it.

Our second point concerns the perforating veins. We believe the importance of normal perforating veins to have been exaggerated. Firstly, most perforators do not, as commonly supposed, consist of a **single channel of significant size**. Instead, as well as being small to start with, most divide into three or more branches after penetrating the deep fascia; so that the vessels that enter the deep vein are very small indeed (barely visible to the naked eye). According to Poiseuille's law, for a given head of pressure, flow of a Newtonian fluid (blood is not very different) varies as (radius of the vessel)[4]. After having dissected a perforator half the size or one-third the size of the main collecting channel, most of us will rightly guess that they represent a fourth and a ninth of the cross-sectional area of the main vessel respectively. Few of us, however, will realize that the same tributaries possess many times higher resistance to flow than common sense would make us believe. If we take into consideration that there are in all only a few dozen perforators, it is evident that of the blood in a saphenous vein only a fraction of one per cent would be expected to go via normal perforators.

Our next point concerns **retrograde** flow. The idea that valvular incompetence can cause continuous retrograde flow in superficial veins, while flow in deep veins is simultaneously continuing in the normal direction is mistaken. In fact, it would be a mechanical impossibility. Real retrograde flow is only possible momentarily during activation of an accessory pump. Much apparent retrograde flow, in relation to the leg, is not really retrograde in relation to the heart.

Our third point concerns the time **taken for the full picture of chronic venous insufficiency**—even an ulcer—to develop. Ulcers are often post-phlebitic and are then assumed to have been the result of loss of carrying capacity. In our view this is a mistake, for it is **after**, not before compensatory dilatation of other veins has occurred that the trophic changes develop. It would seem evident to us, therefore, that it is not loss of carrying capacity, but increased carrying capacity that causes them. How could this be? We can suggest an explanation. It lies in what we have named 'preferred routes'. Blood from capillaries has a great many alternative routes via veins. **Which ones it chooses is not a matter of chance.** The proportion of blood going by each route is bound to be in inverse proportion to its share of the total resistance. Thus a route which becomes dilated will take a disproportionately larger fraction than previously. A route which became twice as wide as an alternative one could be expected to carry 20 or 30 times the proportion of blood and the previous route would become starved (as in the subclavian steal syndrome).

These can start at the level of very small veins or even at the level of arterio-venous capillaries. And it is these capillaries which, we suggest, when dilated constitute the arterio-venous anastomoses of Piulachs and Vidal-Barraquer (1953) and others, and which account for the well-known increased oxygen saturation and greater warmth of varicose-vein blood, and the diminished capillary time of Lipiodol injected into the arteries at phlebography.

All this can be reversed, and the circulation 'normalized' by excising **all** the dilated 'preferred routes' or, as we call the visible ones, the 'pathological circuits'. So we conclude by saying that on theoretical grounds the therapy for varicose veins—a condition consisting of more or less extensive, but **always regional** dilatation of segments of the superficial venous network—should be aimed at a **complete and permanent** removal of these dilated segments. In practical terms this means even for skilled surgeons an operation which takes an average of two hours. But the results, particularly if evaluated on a long-term basis, are so rewarding that this time is fully justified.

References

Aird, I. (1957). *A Companion in Surgical Studies*. Second ed. E. & S. Livingstone Ltd., Edinburgh and London.

Allenby, F., Pflug., J. J., Boardman, L. and Calnan, J. S. (1973). Effects of external pneumatic intermittent compression on fibrinolysis in man. *The Lancet*, **ii**, 1412–1414.

Aukland, K. (1973). Autoregulation of interstitial-fluid volume. Edema-preventing mechanisms. *Scand. J. clin. Lab. Invest.*, **31**, 247.

Barron, D. H. (1960). In *Medical Physiology and Biophysics*, ed. Ruch, T. C. and Fulton, J. F. Eighteenth edn. W. B. Saunders Co., Philadelphia and London.

Basmajian, J. V. (1952). Distribution of valves in the femoral, external iliac, and common iliac veins and their relationship to varicose veins. *Sur. Gynec. & Obstet.*, **95**, 537–542.

Bassi, G. (1956). Rôle des anastomoses artério-veineuses dans la pathologie variqueuse. *Presse méd.*, **64**, 1264–1265.

Bauer, G. (1948). The etiology of leg ulcers and their treatment by resection of the popliteal vein. *J. internat. Chir.*, **8**, 937.

Bayliss, W. M. and Starling, E. H. (1894). Observations on venous pressures and their relationship to capillary pressures. *J. Physiol.*, **16**, 159–202.

Bevegård, B. S. and Shepherd, J. T. (1967). Regulation of the circulation during exercise in man. *Physiol. Rev.*, **47**, 178–213.

Blalock, A. (1929). Oxygen content of blood in patients with varicose veins. *Arch. Surg.*, **19**, 898–909.

Bryant, M. F., Lazenby, W. D. and Howard, J. M. (1958). Experimental replacement of short segments of veins. *Arch. Surg.*, **76**, 289–293.

Burkitt, D. P. (1972). Varicose veins, deep vein thrombosis, and haemorrhoids: epidemiology and suggested aetiology. *Brit. med. J.*, **2**, 556–561.

Calnan, J. S., Ford, P. M., Holt, P. J. and Pflug, J. J. (1972). Implanted tissue cages—a study in rabbits. *Brit. J. plast. Surg.*, **25**, 164–174.

Calnan, J. S., Pflug, J. J., Reis, N. D. and Taylor, L. M. (1970). Lymphatic pressures and the flow of lymph. *Brit. J. Plastic Surg.*, **XXIII**, No. 4, 305–317.

Casley-Smith, J. R. (1970). Lymphatic fine structure in the formation of lymph. *Forum Medici*, **12**, 8–23. (Publ. Zyma S.A., Nyon, Switzerland.)

Crockett, D. J. (1956). The protein levels of oedema fluids. *The Lancet*, **ii**, 1179–1182.

Daniel, D. G. (1969). Estrogens and puerperal thromboembolism. *Amer. Heart J.*, **78**, 720–722.

Dodd, H. and Cockett, S. B. (1956). In *The Pathology and Surgery of the Veins of the Leg*. Longmans, Edinburgh and London.

Fegan, W. G. Anatomy and pathophysiology of varicose veins. In *Venous Diseases—Medical and Surgical Management*.
Proceedings of American European Symposium on Venous Diseases, Montreux 1974. Foundation International Cooperation in the Medical Sciences, Montreux, Switzerland. 1974.

Fowler, H. W. (1965). *Modern English Usage*. Second edn., revised by Sir Ernest Gowers. Clarendon Press, Oxford.

Gordon-Smith, I. C., Grundy, D. J., Le Quesne, L. P., Newcombe, J. F. and Bramble, F. J. (1972). Controlled trial of two regimens of subcutaneous heparin in prevention of postoperative deep-vein thrombosis. *The Lancet*, **i**, 1133–1135.

Gosling, R. G., King, D. H., Newman, D. L., Taylor, G. and Weindling, A. M. (1972). In *Blood Flow Measurement*, ed. Roberts, V. C. Chapter 5: Measurement of aortic elasticity by ultrasound and its relevance to atherogenesis. Sector Publishing Ltd., London.

Guyton, A. C. (1963). A concept of negative interstitial pressure based on pressures in implanted perforated capsules. *Circ. Res.*, **12**, 399–414.

Guyton, A. C., Armstrong, G. G. and Crowell, J. W. D. (1960). Negative pressure in interstitial spaces. *Physiologist*, **3**, 70.

Guyton, A. C., Granger, H. J. and Taylor, A. E. (1971). Interstitial fluid pressure. *Physiol. Rev.*, **51**, 527–562.

Haeger, K. (1968). The treatment of varicose veins in pregnancy by radical operation or conservatively. *Acta Obstet. Gynec. Scand.*, **47**, 233–246.

Haeger, K. M. and Lindell, S.-E. (1966). Oxygen tension in blood from varicose veins. *J. cardiovasc. Surg.*, **7**, 69–73.

Hills, N. H., Pflug, J. J., Jeyasingh, K., Boardman, Lynn and Calnan, J. S. (1972). Prevention of deep vein thrombosis by intermittent pneumatic compression of calf. *Brit. med. J.*, **2**, 31–135.

Johnson, H. D. (1964). Venous pressure: its physiology and pathology in haemorrhage, shock, and transfusion. *Brit. J. Surg.*, **51**, 276.

Johnson, H. D. (1967). Letter: 'Critical closing pressure'. *Nature*, **215**, 858.

Johnson, H. D. (1973a). Letter: 'Traveller's ankle'. *Brit. med. J.*, **3**, No. 5871, 109.

Johnson, H. D. (1973a). Letter: 'Traveller's ankle'. *Brit. med. J.*, **4**, No. 5887, 300.

Johnson, H. D. (1973c). Letter: 'Traveller's ankle'. *J. amer. med. Assoc.*, **225**, No. 12, 1532–1533.

Kinmonth, J. B. (1954). Lymphangiography in clinical surgery and particularly in treatment of the lymphoedema. Hunterian lecture. *Ann. Roy Coll. Surg. Engl.*, **15**, 300–315.

Lagrue, G., Weil, B., Menard, J. and Milliez, P. (1971). Le syndrome d'œdèmes cycliques idiopathiques. I: Etude clinique. *J. Urol. Nephrol. (Paris)*, **77**, 929–935.

Leak, L. V. (1970). Electron microscopic observations on lymphatic capillaries and the structural components of the connective tissue-lymph interface. *Microvascular Research*, **2**, 361–391.

Linton, R. R. (1938). The communicating veins of lower leg and operative technique for their ligation. *Ann. Surg.*, **107**, 582–593.

Linton, R. R. and Hardy, I. B., Jr. (1948). Postthrombotic syndrome of the lower extremity; treatment by interruption of the superficial femoral vein and ligation and stripping of the long and short saphenous veins. *Surgery*, **24**, 452–468.

Lodin, A. and Lindvall, N. (1961). Congenital absence of valves in the deep veins of the leg: a factor in venous insufficiency. I. Clinical observations; II. Roentgenologic investigations. *Acta dermatovener. (Stockh.)*, **41**, (Suppl. 45), 1–83.

Melrose, D. G. (1972). Personal communication.

Nichol, J., Girling, F., Jerrard, W., Claxton, E. B., and Burton, A. C. (1951). Fundamental instability of the small blood vessels and critical closing pressures in vascular beds. *Amer. J. Physiol.*, **164**, 330–344.

Palma, E. C. and Espéron, R. (1959). Tratamiento del sindrome post-tromboflebitico mediante transplante de safena interna. *Angiologia*, **11**, 87–94.

Palma, E. C. and Espéron, R. (1960). Vein transplants and grafts in the surgical treatment of the postphlebitic syndrome. *J. cardiov. Surg.*, **1**, 94–107.

Pappenheimer, J. R. (1953). Passage of molecules through capillary walls. *Physiol. Rev.*, **33**, 387–423.

Pflug, J. J. (1965a). M.D. Thesis. Charles University, Prague—Medical Academy, Magdeburg. Copy in Library, Royal Postgraduate Medical School, London. German.

Pflug, J. J. (1965b). Prophylaxe der tödlichen Embolien in der Chirurgie mit besonderer Berücksichtigung der Primärthrombosen. *Langenbecks Arch. Klin. Chir.*, **313**, 57–61.

Piulachs, P. and Vidal-Barraquer, F. (1953). Pathogenic study of varicose veins. *Angiology*, **4**, 59–100.

Roberts, V. C. (1972). *Blood Flow Measurement.* Sector Publishing Ltd., London.

Rushmer, R. F. (1961). In *Cardiovascular Dynamics.* Second edn. W. B. Saunders Co., Philadelphia and London.

dos Santos, J. C. (1948). Sur quelques veritès premières oubliées ou méconnues de l'anatomo-physiologie normale et pathologique du système veineux. *Amatus lusitanus*, **7**, 5–33.

Sharnoff, J. G., Kass, H. H. and Mistica, B. A. (1962). A plan of heparinization of the surgical patient to prevent postoperative thromboembolism. *Surg. Gynec. & Obstet.*, **115**, 75–79.

Sigg, K. (1963). Varikosis und Thrombose bei Schwangerschaft, Geburt und Wochenbett. *Zbl. Gynäk.*, **85**, 254–260.

Starling, E. H. (1896). On the absorption of fluid from the connective tissue spaces. *J. Physiol.,* **19**, 312.

Starling, E. H. (1909). *The Fluids of the Body.* W. T. Kreemer & Co., Chicago.

Svejcar, J. Prerovsky, I. and Linhart, J. (1961). Chemical composition of the venous wall of the lower limbs. *Cor Vasa,* **3**, 90–97.

Thompson, N. (1971). Surgical treatment of chronic lymphoedema of the arm and leg. *Brit. J. hosp. Med.,* **5**, 395–408.

Van der Molen, H. R. (1962). 'Ausgewählte Phlebologische Neudrucke.' Edition Varitex, Haarlem, Holland. (German and French in one edition.)

Weber, –. (Reference as given by Bayliss and Starling): 'Ueb. die Anwendung der Wellenlehre auf die Lehre vom Kreislaufe des Blutes'. Reprinted in Ostwald's *Klassiker der exacten Wissenschaften,* p. 30 (from Berichte ü. d. Verhandl. der königl. Sächs. Gesellschaft der Wiss. z. Leipzig, 1850).

Wiederhielm, C. A., Stromberg, D. D. and Lee, D. R. (1970). Oncotic pressure in minute fluid samples and tissues. *Federation Proc.,* **29**, 319 Abs.

Yoffey, J. M. and Courtice, F. C. (1970). *Lymphatics, Lymph and the Lymphomyeloid Complex.* Academic Press, London and New York.